Asthma

Raymond G. Slavin, MD, MACP
St. Louis University School of Medicine

Robert E. Reisman, MD, MACP
State University of New York at Buffalo School of Medicine
Buffalo Medical Group

A|C|P

AMERICAN COLLEGE OF PHYSICIANS
PHILADELPHIA

Clinical Consultant: David R. Goldmann, MD
Acquisitions Editor: Mary K. Ruff
Manager, Book Publishing: David Myers
Developmental Editor: Vicki Hoenigke
Production Supervisor: Allan S. Kleinberg
Editorial Coordinator: Alicia Dillihay
Interior Design: Kate Nichols
Cover Design: Elizabeth Swartz
Index: Nelle Garrecht

Manufactured in the United States of America
Composition by UB Communications
Printing/binding by Versa Press

American College of Physicians (ACP) became an imprint of the American College of Physicians–American Society of Internal Medicine in July 1998.

Library of Congress Cataloging-in-Publication Data

Asthma / [edited by] Raymond G. Slavin, Robert E. Reisman.
   p. ; cm. – (ACP key diseases series)
   Includes bibliographical references and index.
   ISBN 1-930513-29-1
   1. Asthma—Handbooks, manuals, etc. I. Slavin, Raymond G. II. Reisman, Robert E.
III. American College of Physicians–American Society of Internal Medicine. IV. Series.
   [DNLM: 1. Asthma—diagnosis. 2. Asthma—therapy. WF 553 A85114 2002]
RC591.A723 2002
616.2'38—dc21

                       2001053347

The authors have exerted reasonable efforts to ensure that drug selection and dosage set forth in this volume are in accord with current recommendations and practice at the time of publication. In view of ongoing research, occasional changes in government regulations, and the constant flow of information relating to drug therapy and drug reactions, the reader is urged to check the package insert for each drug for any change in indications and dosage and for added warnings and precautions. This care is particularly important when the recommended agent is a new or infrequently used drug. ACP–ASIM is not responsible for any accident or injury resulting from the use of this publication.

02 03 04 05 06/9 8 7 6 5 4 3 2 1

Contributors

Emil J. Bardana, Jr., MD, FACP
Professor of Medicine
Division of Allergy and Clinical
  Immunology
Oregon Health Sciences University
Portland, Oregon

Paula J. Busse, MD
Instructor
Mount Sinai Hospital
Department of Adult Allergy and
  Immunology
New York, New York

William W. Busse, MD, FACP
Professor of Medicine
University of Wisconsin Medical
  School
Madison, Wisconsin

Tammy Heinly, MD
Clinical Associate Professor of
  Internal Medicine and
  Pedriatrics
University of Tennessee College of
  Medicine
Memphis, Tennessee

James T. Li, MD, FACP
Professor of Medicine
Mayo Clinic and Foundation
Rochester, Minnesota

Phillip L. Lieberman, MD, FACP
Clinical Professor of Medicine
Division of Allergy and
  Immunology
University of Tennessee College of
  Medicine
Cordova, Tennessee

Richard F. Lockey, MD, FACP
Professor of Medicine, Pediatrics,
  and Public Health
University of South Florida
  College of Medicine
Department of Internal Medicine
Joy McCann Culverhouse
  Professor in Allergy and
  Immunology
Director, Division of Allergy and
  Immunology
James A. Haley Veterans Hospital
Tampa, Florida

Anthony Montanaro, MD, FACP
Professor and Chairman
Division of Allergy and Clinical
  Immunology
Oregon Health Sciences University
Portland, Oregon

Harold S. Nelson, MD
Senior Staff Physician
Department of Medicine
National Jewish Medical and
  Research Center
Professor of Medicine
University of Colorado Health
  Science Center
Denver, Colorado

Mark T. O'Hollaren, MD
Clinical Professor of Medicine
Oregon Health Sciences University
Portland, Oregon

Thomas A.E. Platts-Mills, MD
Professor
Department of Medicine
Chief
Division of Allergy
University of Virginia Medical
  Center
Charlottesville, Virginia

**Nina C. Ramirez, MD, FAAP,
  FCCP**
Fellow in Training
Department of Internal Medicine
Division of Allergy and
  Immunology
University of South Florida
  College of Medicine
VA Medical Center
Tampa, Florida

Robert E. Reisman, MD, MACP
Clinical Professor of Medicine and
  Pediatrics
State University of New York at
  Buffalo School of Medicine
Buffalo Medical Group
Williamsville, NY

Saba Samee, MD
Fellow in Training
Division of Allergy
University of Virginia Medical
  Center
Charlottesville, Virginia

Michael Schatz, MD, MS, FACP
Kaiser-Permanente
Professor of Medicine
University of California - San
  Diego
San Diego, California

Raymond G. Slavin, MD, MACP
Professor of Internal Medicine
St. Louis University School of
  Medicine
St. Louis, Missouri

**Donald D. Stevenson, MD,
  FACP**
Senior Consultant
Division of Allergy, Asthma, and
  Immunology
Scripps Clinic and the Scripps
  Research Institute
La Jolla, California
Professor of Medicine
University of California - San
  Diego
San Diego, California

**Demetrios S. Theodoropoulos,
  MD, DSc**
Marshfield Clinic - Marshfield
  Center
Marshfield, Wisconsin

Contents

Introduction

O ver the past 20 years asthma has been diagnosed with increasing frequency and is now recognized as a major medical problem in the United States. From 1980 to 1994 asthma prevalence increased by 75% among all race, sex, and age groups (1). In 1998 there were approximately 17 million Americans with asthma, with 12.6 million being adults (2). Combined direct and indirect costs have increased to more than $10.7 billion per year (3). Emergency room visits for asthma are over 1.6 million per year and hospitalizations are nearly 500,000 per year. For asthmatics older than 18 years, 8 million work days are lost annually at a cost of $1.3 billion.

Although deaths from asthma are relatively rare, there has been a substantial increase in recent decades. According to the National Heart, Lung, and Blood Institute, the average age-adjusted death rate due to asthma rose from 0.93 deaths per 100,000 cases between 1979 and 1980 to 1.49 deaths per 100,000 cases between 1993 and 1995 (4). More than 2500 adults in the United States die from asthma each year. Patterns of mortality differ greatly between racial and ethnic groups, with death rates for blacks and Hispanics being 3 to 5.5 times that for whites.

Faced with these facts indicating the tremendous impact of asthma on society, there seemed to us a need for a book on this disease for the practicing internist who will, after all, be caring for the majority of adults with asthma. Our intent was to make this book readable, concise, and eminently practical. As a way of bringing this material into the office setting, the book would feature illustrative case histories. The authors would be allergists certified in internal medicine, members of internal medicine departments, and, most importantly, physicians in touch with the daily needs of the practicing internist.

It was felt that such a work would fit perfectly into the ACP Key Disease series. As with the other books in the series, *Asthma* addresses the disease from a viewpoint of pathogenesis, evaluation, and management. Its 14 chapters provide essential information on the causes and classifications of asthma and its diagnosis and treatment:

- Our understanding of the pathogenesis of asthma has increased substantially in recent years. Paula Busse from Mount Sinai Hospital in New York and William Busse from the University of Wisconsin provide an excellent summary of this topic in Chapter 1. Next, the editors provide an overview of the clinical evaluation and management of asthma that is the basis for the more detailed specific issues subsequently discussed (Chapter 2).

- A number of medical conditions may simulate or be confused with asthma. Likewise, asthma is often underdiagnosed when patient symptoms are not typical. Tammy Heinly and Phillip Lieberman from the University of Tennessee lead us deftly through the differential diagnosis of asthma, stressing those conditions particularly appropriate in the adult asthmatic (Chapter 3).

- Exacerbations of asthma are quite common and may lead to emergency room visits and hospitalizations. The management of acute asthma, stressing both the treatment of acute symptoms and the early treatment of exacerbations that may prevent progression to more acute symptoms, is discussed in Chapter 4 by Nina Ramirez and Richard Lockey from the University of South Florida.

- Chronic asthma management can be generally divided into three areas. The first, perhaps the most ignored, is environmental control, which defines guidelines for minimizing allergen and irritant exposure. This topic is covered by Saba Samee and Thomas Platts-Mills from the University of Virginia (Chapter 5). James Li of the Mayo Clinic next discusses pharmacotherapy, stressing how the focus of asthma treatment has moved from control of bronchospasm to regulation of inflammation (Chapter 6). Finally, Harold Nelson of the National Jewish Medical and Research Center and the University of Colorado deals with the third approach to asthma management, allergen immunotherapy (Chapter 7).

- We then move to special topics that are particularly important for many adult asthmatics. Exercise is a major trigger of asthma, one which generally proves a limiting factor in the patient's daily life. Asthma may limit normal daily exercise or may be a problem particularly during strenuous activities such as competitive sports. Mark O'Hollaren from Oregon Health Sciences University writes about the diagnosis and management of this condition (Chapter 8).

- There is increased evidence that important relationships exist between the upper and lower airways. One of the editors, Raymond Slavin from St. Louis University, explores the basis for treatment of upper airway disease, namely rhinitis and sinusitis, which may have beneficial effects on asthma (Chapter 9).

- Asthma in the pregnant patient offers particular problems to both the mother and fetus. Michael Schatz of Kaiser Permanente and the University of California in San Diego offers a safe and practical approach to this problem in Chapter 10.

- The elderly patient is being increasingly diagnosed with asthma. Anthony Montanaro from the University of Oregon deals with this population of patients and the particular problems they may have in terms of both associated disease processes and medications that can influence asthma (Chapter 11).

- Much attention has been paid to the allergen burden in the outside air and in the home. The workplace is also a potentially important area for the asthmatic. Emil Bardana from Oregon Health Sciences University covers the topic of occupational asthma in Chapter 12.

- It has been said that America has become a nation of pill takers. Donald Stevenson from the Scripps Clinic and the University of California in San Diego discusses how medications taken for other medical conditions may unfavorably impact on asthma (Chapter 13).

- Finally, a common trigger for asthma appears to be gastroesophageal reflux disease, which seems to be occurring in almost epidemic proportions. Demetrius Theodoropoulos from the Marshfield Clinic in Wisconsin describes how to suspect and treat this common condition and elaborates on the relationship between gastroesophageal reflux and the respiratory tract (Chapter 14).

Our intent has been throughout to provide the internist with a practical, concise, readable text on asthma and its treatment. With the aid of our stellar group of authors, we believe we have accomplished this goal. We are grateful to the American College of Physicians-American Society for Internal Medicine for offering us the opportunity to carry out this endeavor. In particular, we thank Mary Ruff for her initiative, enthusiasm, and encouragement.

Raymond G. Slavin
Robert E. Reisman

REFERENCES

1. **Mannino DM, Horne DG, Pertowski CA, et al.** Surveillance for asthma—United States: 1960-1995. MMWR. 1998;47:1–28.
2. **American Lung Association, Epidemiology and Statistics Unit.** Trends in Asthma, Morbidity and Mortality. New York; February 2000.
3. **Weiss KB, Sullivan SD, Lyttle CS.** Trends in the cost of illness for asthma in the United States: 1985-1994. J Allergy Clin Immunol. 2000;106:493–9.
4. **National Institutes of Health, National Heart, Lung, and Blood Institute.** Data Fact Sheet: Asthma Statistics. Bethesda, MD; January 1999.

1

■ ■ ■

Pathogenesis of Asthma

Paula J. Busse, MD

William W. Busse, MD

The diagnosis of bronchial asthma is based upon characteristic symptoms and physiologic manifestations. The initial diagnosis may be difficult because asthma shares some features (e.g., shortness of breath, chest tightness, wheezing) with several other respiratory disorders (see Chapter 3). However, asthma is distinct in that its symptoms usually are reversible either spontaneously or with appropriate treatment. Advances in research over the past decades have shown that these symptoms are secondary to reversible airflow obstruction produced by edema, airway smooth muscle contraction, and inflammation.

The epidemiologic study of bronchial asthma is interesting for several reasons. The prevalence of asthma worldwide has more than doubled in the latter part of the 20th century, placing a large financial burden on health care resources as a result. In the United States, it has been estimated that asthma costs at least 6 billion dollars per year for physician visits, medication, and laboratory evaluation, and over 10.7 billion dollars of costs in days missed from work (1). The number of asthmatic patients worldwide has not increased in a uniform pattern. English-speaking and Western countries tend to have the highest prevalence and fastest growth rates of childhood asthma. For example, Vietnam, Finland, Taiwan, and New Guinea are among the areas of the world with the lowest prevalence of asthma, whereas other countries, including the United States, Scotland, Australia, and New Zealand, tend to have markedly higher rates. In the United States, approximately 5.6% of the United States population, or 15 million people, were known to have asthma in the early 1990s (2). These pockets of asthmatic patients and families allow speculation on the genetic components to this disease (which have been confirmed) and on the possibility that its development, or expression, is influenced by environmental factors associated

1

with "Westernization" of culture, including early sensitization to common allergens, prevention of common childhood infections, and exposure to cigarette smoke.

Not only has there been an increase in asthma prevalence, there has also been a rise in morbidity, with more patients experiencing asthma exacerbations. In the United States, these patients are more likely to be African-Americans from large inner cities. This increase coincides with improved recognition and treatment of asthma. This trend also gives further clues into the pathogenesis of asthma—in particular, environmental causes. In addition, although deaths from asthma are relatively rare, they have increased as well. In the United States alone, it has been estimated that over a 10-year period asthma deaths increased as much as 35% (3).

Natural History

Asthma is primarily a disease of childhood, with half of all asthmatic patients receiving their diagnosis by 3 years of age and 80% by 6 years of age. Making the diagnosis of asthma in infants or children may be rather difficult. Asthma is a disease clinically characterized by wheezing and coughing (especially at night) and confirmed by pulmonary function testing, which is difficult for children under the age of 5 years to perform. In addition, it is not uncommon for young children to wheeze, especially after respiratory syncytial virus (RSV) infections. It has been estimated that about 20% of children develop wheezing with RSV infections, but for most this is only a transient feature. Approximately 15% of patients who wheeze after infection will continue to wheeze past the age of 6 years. Factors that favor persistent wheezing (asthma) include female gender; degree of other atopic (allergic) diseases, including atopic dermatitis, food allergy, and allergic rhinitis; a family history of atopy; exposure to cigarette smoke; poor intrinsic lung function; and severity of symptoms.

Asthma typically begins in childhood with episodes of wheezing. Martinez and colleagues demonstrated that certain other risk factors (i.e., family history, reduced lung function in infancy) may contribute to the development of asthma. In their study, children who wheeze before the age of 3 years and persist at 6 years of age were more likely to have an elevated serum IgE level, have diminished lung functions at 6 years of age, and were born to mothers with a history of asthma. On the other hand, children who had transient wheezing before the age of 3 years, but not after 6 years, were more likely to have a normal serum IgE level, no skin-prick test responses, diminished lung functions only at 1 year of age, and maternal smoke exposure, but no history of asthma (4).

It has been estimated that less than 20% of adults have "outgrown" childhood asthma. One study followed asthmatic patients, initially seen between 8 to 12 years of age, for a mean period of 15 years. During follow-up, patients completed questionnaires, underwent skin testing, performed spirometry, and had measurements of airway hyperresponsiveness. Of these asthmatic children, 76% were symptomatic as adults (women 85%, men 72%) and 54% used asthma medications. The persistence of asthma into adulthood was best predicted by the severity of childhood asthma. Patients who only had mild asthma as a child had a forced expiratory volume in one second (FEV_1) value of normal or near normal as an adult, and those with more severe asthma as a child had a lower FEV_1 value as an adult (5).

Many children may not "outgrow" their asthma but instead develop a period of quiescence and suffer a relapse later in life. Patients who tend to experience asthma relapses in adulthood are more likely to be female, have higher rates of atopy, and have had significant exposure to, typically, first-hand cigarette smoke. Frequently, patients complain of asthma symptoms beginning in adulthood, but upon further questioning it is revealed that they have had childhood asthma. When making the diagnosis of adult-onset asthma, care is necessary to distinguish it from other causes of wheezing and chronic coughing including chronic obstructive pulmonary disease (COPD), gastroesophageal reflux, post-nasal drip from sinusitis, vocal cord dysfunction, and potentially fixed airway obstructions including tumors or nodules on the vocal cord (see Chapter 3).

There are relatively few studies on the influence of early asthma treatment on disease progression. Typically, after the age of 35 years, even nonasthmatic adults will experience a decline of approximately 20 to 25 mL/year of FEV_1, and this rate is felt to be accelerated in asthma. This rate of FEV_1 decline may become so significant that some with adult asthma may eventually experience irreversible airflow obstruction. Short-term studies have shown that anti-inflammatory treatment decreases mortality, rates of hospitalizations, and numbers of exacerbations. Biopsy-proven studies have shown that a treatment regimen including anti-inflammatory medication may also reduce several of the pathologic inflammatory changes seen in asthma. Inhaled steroids specifically target inflammation, whereas beta-agonists do not have the same effect if used alone.

Factors Involved in Asthma Pathogenesis and Severity

The development of asthma is based upon multiple factors, including genetics and environment. The onset of the disease most likely arises from an interaction between genetic and environmental influences or the gene-by-environment response (Fig. 1-1).

Exposure to Allergens

Exposure to both indoor (pets, cockroaches, house dust mite, certain molds—in particular, *Alternaria*) and outdoor allergens (molds) contributes

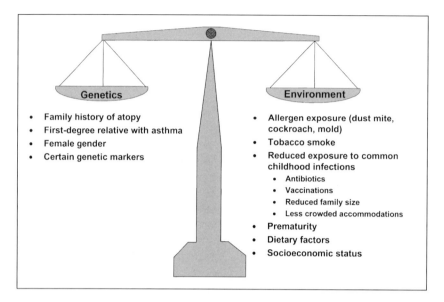

Genetics
- Family history of atopy
- First-degree relative with asthma
- Female gender
- Certain genetic markers

Environment
- Allergen exposure (dust mite, cockroach, mold)
- Tobacco smoke
- Reduced exposure to common childhood infections
  - Antibiotics
  - Vaccinations
  - Reduced family size
  - Less crowded accommodations
- Prematurity
- Dietary factors
- Socioeconomic status

Figure 1-1 Potential factors associated with asthma pathogenesis. The pathogenesis of asthma is thought to be secondary to the interaction between certain genetic *and* environmental factors. The presence of, or exposure to, one or more of these factors may tip the individual towards developing asthma.

to asthma pathogenesis. This may be especially so if exposure occurs early in life. An increased exposure to these allergic antigens at a young age tips the developing immune system to react in an allergic manner. Evidence of allergic sensitization can be suggested by history but is confirmed by positive skin-prick testing or serum levels of IgE.

Much work has been done on the relationship between the indoor allergen, house dust mite, and risk for asthma. Asthma is increased in countries with a higher humidity, an environment preferred by mites. In addition, indoor locations (e.g., upholstery, rugs, stuffed animals, curtains, bedding) provide an appropriate environment for these creatures, and as children spend more time inside the house, exposure to mite antigenic bodies and feces increases. It has been suggested that sensitization via exposure to dust mites during the first two years of life is a significant factor in the development of asthma and may even cause its earlier onset. The German cockroach is another important indoor allergen that is a risk factor for asthma. Unlike dust mites, which typically inhabit the bedroom where the potential for close contact exists, most cockroaches reside in kitchens. Other important indoor allergens include family pets such as cats and dogs. Unlike cockroaches and dust mite particles, their antigens are more likely to be airborne and can travel far. Importantly, in southern parts of the United States exposure to outdoor fungi and the indoor fungi *Alternaria* has been linked to severe asthma.

The "Hygiene Hypothesis"

Recently, it has been hypothesized that certain medical and technological advances in the Western world play important roles in the increase of asthma. In particular, vaccines, purified drinking water, and antibiotics have prevented many of the typical early childhood infections and as a result may tilt the immune system towards an "allergic pathway." The immune system has two arms, based upon the prevalence of specific types of T cells, which can be divided into two types, Th1 and Th2, based upon their cytokine production. Th1 cells produce IL-2, IFN-γ, and TNF-α, which are involved in host defense. Th2 cells secrete IL-3, -4, -5, -6, -10, and -13 to cause allergic inflammation. In humans, T lymphocytes are classified as Th1-like or Th2-like because there may be some crossover production (Fig. 1-2).

In 1989, Strachan and colleagues (6) proposed that infection in early childhood, possibly transmitted by contact with older siblings, or acquired prenatally from a mother infected by contact with her older children will activate the development of the immune system along a Th1-like pathway, and away from a Th2-like pathway, reducing the possibility for development of asthma or allergic disorders. As atopy was decreased in large families, it was hypothesized that as the family grows in size, there is an increased chance of infection, secondary to contact with older siblings or

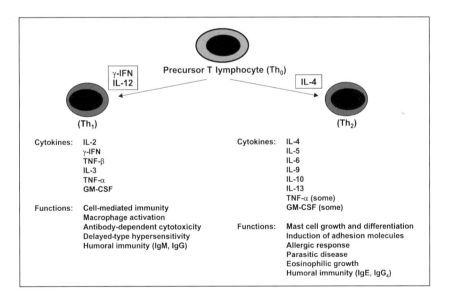

Figure 1-2 Th1 versus Th2 paradigm. Based upon cytokine production in murine models, T lymphocytes may be classified as one of two types: Th1 or Th2. Both of these cell types are derived from a precursor T lymphocyte, Th0, and develop based upon the presence of IFN-γ and/or IL-12 (Th1) or via IL-4 (Th2). Both types have different immune functions, based upon the respective cytokines they secrete. Th1-like cells are typically involved in cell-mediated immunity, whereas Th2-like cells are involved in the allergic response.

prenatally via a mother infected, activating Th1-like cells. Some studies support the "hygiene hypothesis." For example, in a cohort of 262 children in Guinea-Bissau, West Africa, the incidence of measles was inversely related to atopy (7). Similar trends were seen in Air Force students in Italy, where the prevalence of atopy was less common among subjects who were seropositive to hepatitis A (8). Finally, a group of Japanese schoolchildren (9) who received BCG and demonstrated a strong positive tuberculin response (delayed hypersensitivity to *Mycobacterium tuberculosis*) had a lower incidence of asthma and serum IgE levels. In addition, a recently published Finnish study compared patients with a history of active tuberculosis infection with age, sex, and geographically matched controls and found that a history of active tuberculosis infection in childhood significantly reduced the occurrence of subsequent asthma in the female subjects (10).

Although there is much to support the hygiene hypothesis, questions remain. A recent Finnish study failed to find an inverse relationship between a history of measles infection and asthma. In fact, this group, after following children during a four-year period during which a "catch-up" phase for administering the MMR vaccine was given, discovered that more atopic diseases, including asthma, were prevalent among children and adolescents with a history of naturally occurring measles (11). Asthma pathogenesis is, however, multifactorial. It has been demonstrated that infants who attend day care centers before 6 months of age actually had lower incidences of asthma in later childhood. This seems somewhat perplexing because RSV is commonly spread in nurseries and increases the likelihood of post-infectious wheezing. However, it is possible that in certain individuals these infections may shift the development of the immune system away from allergic diseases, whereas other individuals with a genetic predisposition and other potential factors may instead continue to wheeze.

Genetic Factors

Genetics plays a large role in the eventual expression of asthma (Case 1-1). Studies of children from at least one asthmatic parent demonstrate that the asthma phenotype is present in approximately 25% of offspring. In addition, twin studies have found concordance rates for asthma ranging from 4.8% to 33% for dizygotic twins and from 12% to 89% in monozygotic twins.

Interestingly, genetic linkage studies have revealed multiple human chromosomes associated with potential phenotypes of asthma. Human chromosome 5q contains many of the genes associated with production of certain cytokines (IL-3, -4, -5, -9, and -13) linked to airway hyperresponsiveness, to the beta-adrenergic receptor, and to total serum IgE. Linkage to chromosome 6 is associated with eosinophilia; chromosome 11q is linked to the high-affinity IgE receptor found on mast cells and basophils; and chromosome 14q is linked to the T-cell receptor. Because there is an environmental component to asthma pathogenesis that is well accepted, it is likely that

CASE 1-1   *Determining the probability that a child will develop asthma: genetic and environmental factors*

A newly married couple wishes to start a family. The wife has a history of childhood asthma but no longer needs medications for it. However, she has seasonal allergic rhinitis. What is the probability that their child will have asthma? Should they take precautions (e.g., preventing the child from attending day care so that he or she is not exposed early to infections, not having a pet cat) to perhaps prevent the development of asthma in the newborn? What environmental changes can you suggest?

Discussion

A maternal history of asthma, as well as allergic rhinitis, is a significant risk factor for asthma development in the child. Besides these genetic factors, environmental exposures are important. However, it is not recommended that atopically prone children be withheld from day care centers in order to minimize exposure to RSV, which has been associated with development of asthma in children. In fact, some researchers believe that acquisition of early childhood infections may in certain individuals actually sway the immune system to develop into a Th1-like one, and away from allergy. Although studies are not conclusive about prevention of asthma via reduced exposure to family pets, it is generally not a good idea to subject the child to such common allergens. In addition, the family should take precautions against dust mites, because early exposure, even in the nonatopic child, may predispose him or her to asthma. Also avoidance of maternal smoking, even *in utero*, is suggested.

there is a gene-by-environment interaction. Interesting questions remain, however: Do environmental factors trigger genetically predisposed individuals or vice-versa? At what age do genetic factors begin to play a major role?

Respiratory Infections

Many observations have linked certain upper respiratory viral infections—in particular, RSV and, less commonly, parainfluenza—with episodes of transient wheezing and possibly later asthma development. Approximately 1 in 5 infants with RSV wheezes, but only 15% of those who wheeze with a respiratory infection will develop persistent asthma. Why some children who wheeze with infections later develop asthma is unclear, but there are a number of hypotheses. It has been suggested that severe RSV infection produces inflammatory bronchiolitis, potentially leading to airway injury and remodeling. These permanent lung-growth changes may cause the persistent wheezing. Another possibility is that RSV infection, in genetically prone atopic individuals, influences the developing immune system to become more allergic. IgE to RSV has been detected, and individuals infected with RSV may have eosinophilia and markers of eosinophil activation including increased eosinophilic cationic protein. Therefore the RSV infection may be the nidus that tips the development of the immune system towards an allergic predisposition.

RSV infections are *rarely* experienced by adults, because most children have been exposed to RSV by the age of 2 years. However, in adult asthma, other respiratory viral infections—in particular, rhinovirus (RV, the common cold virus)—exacerbate asthma. Unlike RSV, RV has many strains; therefore immunity is not gained by previous exposure, making it a common infection of both older children and adults. By means of RT-PCR, as many as 60% to 75% of wheezing episodes in children and 50% in adults can be induced by RV, but other airway infections, such as influenza and parainfluenza, have also been detected. More recently, *Chlamydia pneumoniae* infection, which has been implicated as an etiology of arteriosclerosis in some patients, has also been targeted as a possible bacteria that may exacerbate or cause asthma.

An interesting question is how RV, an upper airway infection, provokes responses in the lower airway. Experimental work has suggested several possible interactions between the upper and lower airways of the asthmatic subjects infected with RV. One explanation is that RV infections migrate to the lower airways. This has been documented by lower bronchial biopsies of patients experimentally infected with RV. In addition, bronchoalveolar lavage (BAL) specimens from these patients have shown evidence of RV RNA. In addition, it is possible that RV infections may cause an exaggerated response to subsequent antigen or allergen exposure. The upper and lower airways are neurogenically connected. For example, RV in the upper airways could lead to neuropeptide release from sensory C fibers producing bronchospasm or interfere with the release of the brochodilator nitric oxide (NO) produced by nonadrenergic noncholinergic neurons.

The exact mechanism of how respiratory viruses provoke airway inflammation is not fully known. What is known is that viruses replicate within the airway epithelium, leading to secretion not only of additional RV particles but of multiple cytokines and chemokines. Some of the newly replicated RV particles may exit the epithelium and bind to several adhesion molecules, notably ICAM-1 and the low-density lipoprotein receptor, LDLr, located on antigen-presenting cells (APCs) such as macrophages, B cells, and dendritic cells. This interaction produces IFN-γ, IL-12, and IL-18, which in turn together activate either CD4+ T cells or natural killer cells (a type of T cell involved in cytolytic reactions). Other RV particles may be processed by APCs and presented to T cells, typically occurring 7 to 10 days after introduction of the virus, and may be a possible explanation of why patients with asthma may have prolonged wheezing after an upper respiratory viral infection. The activation of the CD4+ T cells, by either mechanism, produces additional cytokines, chemokines, adhesion molecules, and possibly leukotrienes. These mediators can recruit other inflammatory cells to the airways or increase the "leakiness" of the endothelial surfaces, producing transudation of plasma proteins from the vascular endothelial wall to the nasal mucosa, leading to nasal congestion and secretion. Furthermore, release of cytokines can cause airway hyperresponsiveness. Either by direct or indirect activation of the CD4+ cell, it has been proposed that the RV may also cause production of an epithelial growth factor or potentially infect smooth muscles of the airway. Both mechanisms can produce airway hyperresponsiveness and remodeling.

Tobacco Smoke

Environmental tobacco smoke (ETS) exposure alters lung functions in infants and increases the risk for lower respiratory tract illnesses. These processes can predispose the child to asthma. It has been demonstrated that as early as 2 weeks of age *in utero* exposure to ETS predisposes the child towards asthma via changes in the elastic structure of the developing fetal lung. This most likely occurs by vasoconstriction from nicotine that decreases uterine blood flow and produces fetal hypoxia with growth retardation. Passive smoke exposure to infants or children has also been causally associated with an increased risk of lower respiratory tract infections, a small but significant dose-dependent reduction in pulmonary function, and increased severity of asthma symptoms.

Socioeconomic Status

In general, affluent areas of the Western world tend to have a higher prevalence of asthma and other atopic diseases. In developing parts of the world, in contrast, there has been a gradient between affluent and poor regions. For example, in Harare, the capital of Zimbabwe, the prevalence of airway hyperresponsiveness was significantly higher in a wealthier part of the city than in its poorer sections (12). However, these trends do not necessarily follow in the United States, where asthma disproportionately affects minority children living in urban poverty. Some of the largest populations of asthma patients are located in inner-city areas of New York, Baltimore, and Los Angeles. In addition, these patients tend to have higher morbidities and mortalities from their asthma. Several factors have been proposed to account for this trend. One is an increased level of indoor allergens from cockroaches, mice, and other rodents. In addition, it is often difficult for populations of a lower socioeconomic status (SES) to afford certain precautions against dust mites such as protective covers on the bedding. Populations of lower SES also tend to have less access to medical care. As a result, these patients may not receive treatment and preventive measures to control asthma.

Air Pollution and Diesel Exhaust Fuel

Data show that certain air pollutants exacerbate pre-existing asthma but do not necessarily cause allergies and asthma to develop. German reunification several years ago was a perfect model for studying the effect of environmental pollution while controlling for genetic factors. In the former East Germany there was a heavier concentration of industrial pollutants such as SO_2 than in the former West Germany. Since unification, rates of asthma and atopic diseases have increased in the cities of West Germany.

In addition, many people have questioned the effect of the growing ozone layer on the development of asthma. A single exposure to ozone may produce symptoms consistent with asthma, including shortness of breath, wheezing, and possibly depressed FEV_1; however, long-term studies have not shown consistent results.

Diesel exhaust particles modulate the immune system under experimental situations and enhance IgE production.

Diet

The role of maternal diet during pregnancy and breastfeeding in relationship to the development of allergic diseases, in particular asthma, is highly controversial. Although cord blood samples indicate hypersensitivity towards particular foods eaten by the mother during pregnancy, there is no evidence to date that maternal elimination of diets of highly allergenic foods prevents asthma development in newborns. Some studies, however, recommend prolonged breastfeeding to prevent respiratory allergy. One Finnish study examined 150 infants who were grouped according to the duration of breastfeeding and followed to the development of atopic diseases, including asthma, until 17 years of age (13). Breastfeeding for less than 1 month, then switching to cow's milk formula, significantly increased the asthma prevalence of these subjects. However, when compared with a family with a first-degree relative with atopy, hereditary factors had similar significance for asthma development. In general, current studies are difficult to perform and interpret for a number of reasons, including environmental exposures to offending antigens, heredity, maternal diet of potentially highly allergenic foods, type of formula, and progression of solid foods given to the infant. In addition, others have questioned the effect of the child's diet on asthma development, such as the benefits from consumption of fish fatty acids (omega-3) on protection from bronchial hyperreactivity.

Worsening of Symptoms at Nighttime

Asthma symptoms tend to be worse in the peak hours of the morning (typically 4 A.M.) and more quiescent in the early afternoon (between noon and 4 P.M.). This phenomenon is secondary to the circadian rhythm of the body's natural production of cortisol, which has its nadir between midnight and 4 A.M. and peaks from 8 A.M. to noon. It seems that symptoms of asthma lag approximately 4 hours after these circadian shifts. In addition, the circadian cycle is not based upon actual clock time but rather on the person's sleep-wake cycle. Cortisol will typically suppress inflammatory cells by several known (i.e., interference of cytokine production, acceleration of apoptosis) and unknown mechanisms. Asthmatic patients may also have worsening of symptoms at night secondary to postnasal drip from allergic rhinitis or sinusitis that can cause irritation of the bronchial tree. In addition, gastroesophageal reflux, which may be exacerbated as the patient lies down, may worsen asthma. Also, bedding tends to be a nice home for dust mites and allows for close contact between an allergen and a sensitized patient, which may also worsen the patient's asthma systems as he or she lies on pillows and bedding.

Cellular Inflammation in Asthmatic Airways

We now recognize that factors of airway inflammation exist in asthmatic subjects. Initial appreciation of inflammation stemmed from autopsies of patients with acute fatal attacks. With the use of fiberoptic bronchoscopy, it is possible to biopsy patients with asthma, even its severe variety. From these studies, it is possible to characterize which inflammatory cells are associated with asthma and how these cells may contribute to it.

Inflammatory Cells in Asthma

The cellular processes in asthma are apparently well orchestrated and involve several different inflammatory cells and mediators. These inflammatory cells arise from the bone marrow from a noncommitted white blood cell, which has on its surface a particular protein, CD34+. Through specific targeting and developmental pathways, CD34+ cells become a precursor either to a lymphocyte lineage or to granulocytes (eosinophils, neutrophils, basophils, monocytes). Each type of inflammatory cell can play a role in inflammation in asthma.

Mast Cells

Mast cells are the principal effector cells of immediate-type hypersensitivity. They express abundant amounts of a receptor for the IgE antibody on their surfaces to bind preformed IgE with repeated exposure to this antigen. The attached IgE molecule binds the antigen and bridges another, triggering the mast-cell IgE to mediator release. Many mediators are released in 1 to 5 minutes as they are stored preformed (histamine, tryptase, heparin, and, in some mast cells, chymase, carboexpeptidase, and cathepsin G) or generated and then secreted, including LTC_4, after activation synthesis (including LTC_4, PGD_2, and cytokines including TNF-α, IL-4, -5, -6, IL-13; however, this production is minimal compared to that by lymphocytes). In addition, mast cells may cause structural changes via production of laminin,

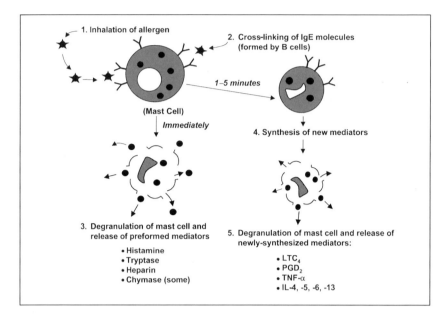

Figure 1-3   Role of the mast cell in asthma. The mast cell is central to the pathogenesis of asthma. It synthesizes and secretes several mediators that produce the typical symptoms of the asthmatic response including bronchoconstriction and edema of the airways. Mast cells are triggered to release these substances via binding of an allergen to its receptor on IgE antibodies, coating the mast cell surface. Upon antigen binding, bridges are formed between the IgE molecules, triggering intracellular events that release the mediators of the mast cell.

collagen IV, and activation of fibroblasts. These mediators produce multiple symptoms common to allergic and asthmatic reactions. For example, histamine will cause bronchoconstriction of the airways, leakiness of the capillaries leading to fluid accumulation in the lungs and tissues, and irritation of nerve fibers producing itch, among many other functions. Many of the prostaglandins produce vasoconstriction of the bronchial tree and leakiness of the capillaries (Fig. 1-3).

T Lymphocytes

The T lymphocytes are key cells in asthma and act to coordinate the actions of the other immune cells, notably the B lymphocytes and eosinophils, and to amplify the production of other immune cells such as the neutrophil, macrophage, mast cell, and dendritic cells via production of cytokines. T lymphocytes are subdivided by the presence of the cell surface marker into either CD4+ or CD8+ cells. Each specific T lymphocyte has its own role. In general, CD4+ cells amplify humoral immunity (antibody production by B lymphocytes) and are referred to as *helper T-cells*. In addition, CD4+ cells recognize foreign antigens that have been processed and presented to them by other cells. This makes CD4+ T lymphocytes pivotal in the pathogenesis of inflammation.

To date, more than 20 cytokines, each with different roles regarding cellular proliferation and recruitment, have been identified. Th1-like cells secrete cytokines involved in delayed-type hyperimmunity (such as seen with tuberculosis infection), whereas Th2-like cells secrete cytokines (IL-3, -4, -5, -6, -10, -13) that are primarily involved in the typical allergic response (see Fig. 1-2). IL-3 stimulates mast cell development in tissues; IL-4 and IL-13 stimulate IgE production, the allergic antibody; IL-5 produces eosinophil maturation; and IL-10 can inhibit many of the macrophage functions as well as increase survival of mast cells. Although both the Th1 and Th2 cells arise from the same CD4+ naïve cells, the presence of IL-12 or IFN-γ presence directs Th1 development, and IL-4 and IL-13 directs Th2 subset development.

The cytokine profile produced by atopic (allergic) individuals from T-cell clones has demonstrated predominantly IL-4 and minimal IFN-γ secretions when exposed to specific antigens. *In vivo* work supports the concept that patients with atopic asthma have a predilection toward Th2-like cells; for example, asthma BAL studies find an increased number of cells expressing mRNA for IL-2, -3, -4, -5, and GM-CSF. In addition, bronchial biopsies reveal a predominant Th2-like cytokine profile. The Th1/Th2 paradigm has become of considerable importance in the study of asthma development. Considerable effort is directed toward study to determine in childhood illnesses how early exposure to allergic antigens may direct the development towards a Th2-like profile.

B Lymphocytes

B lymphocytes produce antibodies, of which there are five broad classifications (IgA, IgG, IgM, IgD, and IgE), each having distinct functions. IgE antibody has classically been thought of as the allergic antibody, and each IgE antibody will have specificity towards one antigen. B lymphocytes become committed to produce specific antibodies, such as IgE, after antigen exposure but only after direct interaction with CD4+ T lymphocytes, which produce IL-4 and IL-13. Upon subsequent antigenic exposure, and with the help of other cytokines, namely IL-2, -5, -6, and TNF-α, these B cells and their progeny produce specific IgE antibodies. Once released by the B cell, IgE molecules attach to high-affinity receptors located on the surfaces of mast cells and basophils, or possibly to low affinity receptors on eosinophils.

Eosinophils

Eosinophilia is a common feature of atopic diseases, including asthma, and is often in proportion to disease severity. Ninety-nine percent of eosinophils reside in tissues to which they are attracted by cytokines (e.g., IL-5) and chemokines (e.g., RANTES and eotaxin). In tissues with active inflammation, the eosinophil life is prolonged by the cytokines IL-5 and GM-CSF.

The role of the eosinophil in asthma is, at present, somewhat unclear. The eosinophil contains several granules with mediators and proteases, of which major basic protein (MBP) makes up the majority. MBP can damage airway epithelium and increase airway responsiveness. In addition, there are other toxins in the granules of the eosinophil, including eosinophil cationic protein (ECP), eosinophil neurotoxin (EDN), and eosinophil peroxidase (EPO), of which the last can use bromide to form hypobromous acid, a toxic metabolite that, together with the cationic proteins, accounts for much of the tissue toxicity and antibacterial and antiparasitic effects associated with degranulation of eosinophils. Eosinophils can produce a large number of cytokines including IL-1, -2, -3, -4, -5, -6, -10, -12, TGF-β, TNF-α, GM-CSF, and macrophage inflammatory protein (MIP)-1α, all of which can be involved with recruitment of other inflammatory cells to the lung. The eosinophil may also produce chemokines, including RANTES, which may activate T lymphocytes and degranulate basophils.

Corticosteriods are the mainstay of asthma management and can inhibit eosinophil migration and survival, most likely via interference with cytokine production by the lymphocytes. In early clinical trials, an antibody directed against IL-5 has been found to decrease circulating IL-5 levels and reduce eosinophil numbers. Despite the suppression of eosinophils in asthmatic patients given anti-IL-5, no improvement in asthma symptoms occurred. This finding has raised some questions regarding the exact importance of the eosinophil in asthma.

Basophils

For many years, basophils were considered to be a circulating form of mast cells. Although these two cell lines share many features, basophils are not mast cells, suggesting a different lineage. More recent work has suggested that basophils and eosinophils come from a common precursor cell. The role of the basophil in the pathogenesis of asthma remains unclear. Elevated basophil numbers have been detected in the sputum and BAL fluids of asthmatics when compared with control subjects. Unlike many of the other inflammatory cells, however, notably the eosinophil or mast cell, the basophil presence may or may not be related to airway hyperresponsiveness.

Neutrophils

The principal biological role of polymorphonuclear leukocytes (PMNs) centers on defense against bacterial infections. These cells contain granule proteases, hydrolases, microbicidal proteins, and enzymes to digest the bacteria, as well as phagocytic capability, and as a result are among the first cells recruited in a bacterial infection. In addition, PMNs can synthesize several cytokines: TNF-α, IL-1, -3, -6, -8, GM-CSF, and G-CSF, which may play roles in defense against bacterial infections or cause inflammation in asthma. In patients dying from acute asthmatic exacerbations, neutrophil accumulation in the airway is a characteristic early picture. Furthermore, in patients with so-called steroid-resistant asthma, a form of asthma refractory to traditional steroid therapy, neutrophils are increased and likely contribute to airway injury.

Epithelial Cells

Originally, epithelial cells were thought to act simply as a nonspecific barrier to toxic and infectious agents of the airway muscle. We now know that they serve other critical functions including secretion of proinflammatory mediators, presentation of foreign particles (antigens), and alteration of the bronchial smooth muscle tone. Among the many cytokines and chemokines produced by epithelial cells are RANTES, eotaxin, IL-8, -16, MCP-1, -3, -4, and MIP-1α. These chemokines are of particular importance in the pathogenesis of asthma because they can cause recruitment of other inflammatory cells. In addition, other inflammatory mediators are produced including nitric oxide, reactive oxygen species, prostaglandins, epithelial growth factor (EGF), and platelet-activating factor.

Dendritic Cells

Dendritic cells line several of the mucosal surfaces as well as the respiratory epithelium. Their major role is to present antigens to other cells such as T lymphocytes. Dendritic cells engulf organisms and, in addition, have dendrites (small arms) on their surface to allow them to travel throughout the body. This ability to travel is extremely valuable because dendritic cells can bring antigens from the respiratory airway and direct them, along with cytokine and chemokines, to lymph nodes where they function as antigen-presenting cells (APCs). In addition, dendritic cells have been found to be the source of several important cytokines such as IFN-γ and IL-12.

Macrophages

Macrophages are constitutive residents of the lung and airways and normally function in host defense mechanisms via their ability to phagocytose organisms and destroy them by the release of reactive oxygen species and lysosomal enzymes. In addition, they play an important role in the inflammatory cascade because they have the ability to secrete several cytokines (IL-1, -6, -8, GM-CSF, TNF-α, and interferons), lipid mediators (TXA_2, LTB_4, LTC_4, LTD_4, and PGD_2), platelet-activating factor, plasminogen activator, several growth factors, and histamine-releasing factor. When activated, they can also secrete matrix metalloproteinases (MMPs) to degrade various extracellular matrix macromolecules including elastin. Furthermore, macrophages act as APCs and reside in the airway. With the introduction of an antigen, macrophages engulf it and present it to T lymphocytes. Macrophages also release several mediators that are involved in inflammation. In addition, macrophages have been demonstrated to have on their cell surface low-affinity IgE receptors, which are increased in patients with atopic asthma and may potentially be involved in mediator release.

Fibroblasts

Fibroblasts retain the ability for growth and regeneration and may eventually develop into smooth muscle cells. Myofibroblasts can then release elastin, fibronectin, and laminin, and produce collagen and reticular elastic fibers as well as proteoglycans and glycoproteins. An increased number of such cells are seen in the asthmatic lung after challenge with antigen.

Airway Response to Antigen

The inflammatory cells described above work in a unique, coordinated fashion to produce the allergic response in asthma. Typically the airway response to antigen is proposed to occur in two phases: the immediate and the late. The early phase of an asthmatic exacerbation usually occurs within 20 to 30 minutes after inhalation of an antigen and is characterized by acute bronchial obstruction. This results from mast-cell activation and effects of its mediators on airway smooth muscle (see Fig. 1-3). Leukotrienes are particularly important because of their profound effects on smooth muscle contraction. Many patients experience a recurrence of bronchial obstruction 4 to 10 hours later, the late-phase reaction (LAR). The LAR is characterized by recruitment of inflammatory cells—notably eosinophils, lymphocytes, and, possibly, basophils—to the airways. These cells are recruited by the production of cytokines and chemokines (e.g., IL-5, RANTES, eotaxin) produced by the stimulated CD4+ cells (Fig. 1-4).

Mechanisms of Cellular Migration

Recently, the mechanisms for recruitment of inflammatory cells to the lungs have become better established. Sequential steps occur, notably activation of the endothelial cells, and eventual rolling of the inflammatory cells along this barrier. Eventually, inflammatory cells are activated, become adherent, and extravasate through the endothelial barrier to reach the lungs. Adhesion molecules on the surfaces of cells and endothelium facilitate this process and can be divided into several types, including selectins, integrins, and members of the immunoglobulin gene superfamilies.

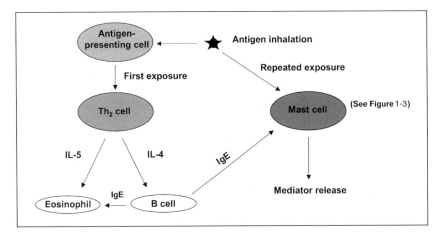

Figure 1-4 Inflammatory cascade in asthma. Upon first introduction to an allergen, the cascade will be recognized by an antigen-presenting cell (APC), typically dendritic cells, macrophages, or B lymphocytes, and engulfed. The APC will process the antigen to a form that can be recognized by the Th2 lymphocyte (in asthma and allergy), which in turn leads to the latter cell producing specific cytokines (e.g., IL-4) that induce IgE production by the B cells. Upon repeated exposure, the same cascade occurs and IL-5 is released, which matures the eosinophils. The antigen may also bind to the preformed IgE molecules that are bound to the mast cell.

Selectins

Selectins are transmembrane glycoproteins whose major function is to assist with "rolling" and loose adherence of inflammatory cells to the endothelial surface. L selectins are found on leukocytes and allow cells to become attracted to, and roll along, the endothelial barrier via nonspecific adhesion. E selectin and P selection are found on the endothelial surfaces and function as the site of attachment of the L selectin. Platelets and endothelium constitutively synthesize P selectin and store it in secretory granules, which are then released upon activation by histamine, thrombin, or reactive oxygen species. E selectin is only produced by endothelial cells and is not stored like P selectin. Instead, E selectin is produced *de novo* upon induction by specific cytokines, lipopolysaccharides, and other inflammatory mediators.

Integrins

Integrins are transmembrane cell-surface proteins that bind to cytoskeletal proteins. They are involved in both cell-cell interactions and cell-substratum adhesion. Integrins, unlike selectins, are only found on leukocytes. To date, only five members have been shown to play a role in leukocyte-endothelial interactions: LFA-1, Mac-1, p150,95, VLA-4, and mucosal-addressing cell adhesion molecule-1 (Md-CAM-1). They play a role in more specific cell adhesion and facilitate chemotaxis.

Immunoglobulin Gene Superfamily

Immunoglobulin gene superfamily adhesion proteins are named because of the presence of immunoglobulin domains. Members of this family are single-chained polypeptides with variable numbers of the immunoglobulin-like extracellular domains. Six members of this group of adhesion proteins have been identified: ICAM-1, -2, -3, VCAM-1, platelet-endothelial cell adhesion marker, and MdCAM-1. ICAM-1 is a marker of B-cell activation and binds to LFA-1.It is constitutively expressed on endothelium, epithelium, and fibroblasts and is up-regulated by many cytokines. ICAM-1 is thought to have a role both in adhesion and migration of leukocytes and is implicated in the later stages of leukocyte migration that require firm adhesion. VCAM-1 is found on endothelial cells and some dendritic cells. VCAM-1 is not constitutively expressed but is readily inducible by IL-1, -4, TNF-α, and LPS. It binds to VLA-4 on eosinophils and lymphocytes. This interaction tends to occur later in the inflammatory migration pathway and is immediately followed by diapedesis of the cells through the adventitia.

Mechanisms of Cellular Migration

The processes of cellular adhesion and selective diapedesis in asthma are complex and involve many of the adhesion molecules described above. In a simplified fashion, inflammatory cells move randomly along the endothelial surface as they are unprimed. Upon stimulation from an inflammatory trigger, the endothelial and leukocyte cells begin to express selectins. This process causes the inflammatory cells to become sticky and roll more slowly. Eventually the leukocyte will skid along the endothelial surface when it encounters a high concentration of inflammatory mediators such as cytokines. This causes an increase in surface-adhesion molecules, and eventually the inflammatory cell will stick to the endothelium. This binding to the endothelium causes the endothelium to loosen its cell-cell interaction, by undefined mechanisms, which then allows the inflammatory cell to migrate into the airway matrix (Fig. 1-5).

In asthma, adhesion molecules are important for cellular recruitment to the airways. Animal models demonstrate that blocking antibodies against certain adhesion molecules can inhibit airway responses as well as the eosinophil influx. In addition, increased levels of VCAM-1, but not ICAM-1 or E selectin, have been demonstrated in tissues from asthmatic subjects. Interestingly, inhaled corticosteroids decrease expression of some of these cell-adhesion molecules.

Airway Remodeling in Asthma

The role of inflammatory cells not only includes defense against bacterial and viral infections but also wound healing. Inflammatory cells are central

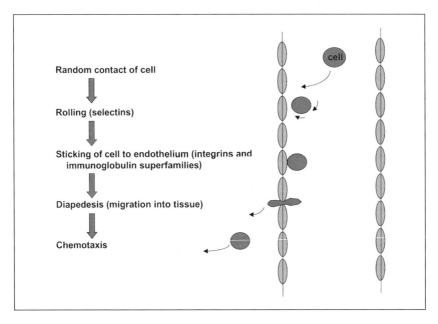

Random contact of cell

Rolling (selectins)

Sticking of cell to endothelium (integrins and immunoglobulin superfamilies)

Diapedesis (migration into tissue)

Chemotaxis

Figure 1-5   Sequence of cellular migration. Inflammatory cells are attracted to sites of inflammation by several types of adhesion molecules that participate in drawing them away from circulation. Cells initially will make random contact with the endothelial surface. However, under the presence of specific cytokines, the inflammatory cells produce adhesion molecules on their surfaces, which makes them slow down and eventually stick to the endothelium. These cells can migrate into the tissue and are drawn to the specific site of inflammation by chemokines.

to the repair of damaged tissue in that they release mediators to recruit other inflammatory cells to the site of injury. These cells release digestive proteases to clean the wound. In addition, fibroblasts are recruited and are essential for deposition of repair tissue, including collagen. Many of these mediators, however, have toxic side effects to mammalian cells.

Asthma is characterized by an excessive concentration of inflammatory cells in the airways. Furthermore, the life span of these inflammatory cells is prolonged in the airways via several growth factors and cytokines (GM-CSF, IL-4, IL-5) that prevent apoptosis or programmed cell death. Cells such as macrophages and eosinophils are particularly responsible for the release of growth factors that may also prolong their own survival. Therefore it is not surprising that chronic inflammation, via release of toxic mediators and subsequent tissue repair, may lead to fixed changes in the airway, including nonreversible obstruction (remodeling) (Fig. 1-6). This hypothesis has been confirmed by analysis of lung biopsies and tissues from autopsies of patients with chronic asthma; irreversible changes in the airways of some patients with chronic asthma have been demonstrated.

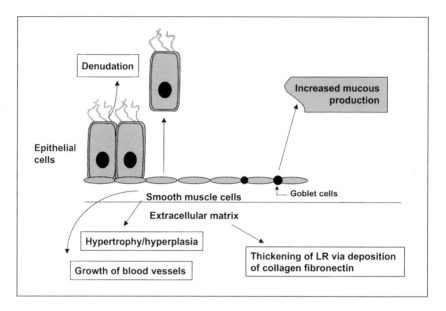

Figure 1-6   Airway remodeling in asthma. The presence of increased inflammatory cells in the asthmatic lung leads to damage in the lung parenchyma that may become permanent. These changes are secondary to the inflammatory mediators released by these cells. Typical pathologic changes include increased smooth muscle mass, thickening of the extracellular matrix, increased mucous glands and production, and denudation of the epithelium. LR = lamina reticularis.

Smooth Muscle

Hypertrophy and hyperplasia of airway smooth muscle have been seen in some asthmatic patients; however, this is not a consistent finding. Muscle enlargement may lead to obstruction and bronchial hyperresponsiveness. Patients dying from asthma exacerbations tend to have increased smooth muscle mass. Much of this smooth muscle hyperplasia and hypertrophy is secondary to cytokines and growth factors produced either by inflammatory cells or the smooth muscle itself. In addition, up-regulation of growth receptors and cell adhesion molecules occurs in the smooth muscle to further this potentially vicious cycle.

Extracellular Matrix

The extracellular matrix (ECM) is a complex structure that serves many functions including a support network of the airways as well as a meshwork that influences the development, migration, and proliferation of many of the inflammatory cell mediators. The ECM can be divided into the basement membrane (BM) and the interstitial matrix (IM). Remodeling in chronic asthma has been well documented in the former.

The basement membrane is composed of two layers: the basal lamina and the lamina reticularis. The thickness of the basal lamina is not affected by asthma. However, a characteristic of asthma is thickening of the lamina reticularis, which may occur early in asthma development. This thickening consists of a deposition of immunoglobulins and/or collagen I, III, IV, and fibronectin, but not laminin. These fibers are produced by activated myofibroblasts.

Remodeling of the interstitial matrix is less well documented. However, certain pathologic changes have been noted in sections of the interstitial matrix. The elastic fibers that comprise the interstitial matrix in asthma appear abnormal and include tangling and increased thickness. Also identified has been an increase of lytic lesions in the elastic fibers. Disruption of the elastic fibers will, in turn, affect the compliance of the asthmatic lung, similar to that seen in emphysema.

Mucous Glands

Excess mucous production is a common feature in chronic asthma. Mucus is normally produced in the human subepithelial glands. In chronic asthma, the increase in mucous secretion appears to be secondary to development of mucus-producing cells that extend into the peripheral bronchioles, where they are normally absent, as well as mucous gland hypertrophy (increase in size). Controversy exists as to whether mucous glands have undergone hyperplasia (increase in numbers), such as is seen in chronic bronchitis. This may be the case in patients dying from acute asthma exacerbations in whom the cause of death includes obstruction of the bronchi by mucus. Autopsies have demonstrated not only an increased size, but *also* number, of goblet cells, but not necessarily in chronic asthma. Animal models have suggested that prolonged allergen exposure may lead to hyperplasia of the mucus-secreting glands. Mucous gland hyperplasia may exist not only in patients with severe asthma and a high potential for mortality but also in patients with milder persistent asthma.

Vascular Dilation and Angiogenesis

Vascular dilation and congestion are central features of inflammation. Dilation of the vessels leads to further leakiness into the lung parachyma, such as is seen in many types of inflammation, and may explain the wheeziness of congestive heart failure. Vascular dilation has been demonstrated in both animal models and human subjects after antigen exposure.

An increase in blood vessels (i.e., angiogenesis) has been reported in chronic asthma. A central part of tissue remodeling is new vessel growth. The exact mechanism that causes new vessel growth remains unclear. Vascular endothelial growth factor or endothelial marker factor VIII levels have not been found to be increased in asthma. However, potential new factors, such as matrix metalloproteinases (MMPs), have been associated with vessel growth and are increased in asthma. Of interest, autopsy studies of patients taking inhaled steroids have shown a decrease in the percentage of vascular area and number of vessels.

Abnormalities in Innervation

The changes in innervation of the remodeled airways have not yet been fully elucidated. However, some studies suggest that a loss of vasoactive intestinal peptide-containing nerves (involved in bronchodilation) may occur as well as an increase in substance P-containing fibers (which leads to bronchodilation). However, these abnormalities are only speculations and have not yet been confirmed.

Clinical Consequences of Airway Remodeling

Nonspecific Bronchial Hyperresponsiveness

Airway remodeling may lead to an increase in bronchial hyperresponsiveness (BHR). Small changes in the airway thickening, as caused by smooth muscle hypertrophy or vascular engorgement, lead to an exaggerated decrease in airway resistance, thus, in turn, causing increases in airway reactivity. In addition, subepithelial collagen deposition can stiffen the inner layer of the airway, increasing the intraluminal airway pressure upon contraction of smooth muscles. Remodeling may also lead to a loss of elastic parenchymal recoil; both factors produce an increased hyperresponsiveness.

Reduced Effect of Bronchodilator Medications

It has been speculated that changes of the smooth muscles, such as hypertrophy and hyperplasia, lead to changes in the velocity of smooth muscle shortening. With normal muscle contraction, actin-myosin cross-bridges form and, as the muscle hypertrophies and grows, these cross-bridges increase in number. As a result, the airway does not relax or stretch with the use of beta-agonists. Therefore it is possible that, with sufficient hypertrophy, beta-agonist therapy will lose effectiveness.

Special Topics

Pathophysiology of Sudden Death from Asthma

Although asthma is considered a chronic airway disease from which patients infrequently die, there are rare asthmatic patients whose history is not significant for frequent exacerbations who suddenly and unexpectedly die. "Typical" asthma deaths (in chronic asthma) occur in patients with a past history of near-fatal attacks who have repeated exposures to or experiences with high concentrations of an offending antigen. Clinically, these patients experience premature airway closure, hyperinflation of the lungs, increased work of breathing, and changes in elastic recoil; as a result, they have significantly depressed expiratory volumes and flow rates. Pathologically, this may arise from widespread inflammation of the airways, typically including eosinophils and neutrophils, airway narrowing from the inflammation and smooth muscle contraction, and airway obstruction from mucosal disruption and the leakage of plasma proteins. In severe cases, there may be evidence of right ventricular strain and compromised left ventricular filling. The typical blood gas pattern initially demonstrates hyperventilation with a low oxygen and CO_2 and resultant respiratory alkalosis, not infrequently accompanied by a metabolic acidosis as well. The severity of the obstruction is reflected by the arterial oxygen tension. As obstruction progresses and respiratory muscle fatigue occurs, CO_2 is retained, and the patient develops respiratory acidosis. Although this may be the pathologic cause of death from chronic asthma, there is a subset of patients with "sudden asphyxic asthma" in whom death occurs after a rapid decompensation and extreme hypercapnia. At autopsy, these patients show more neutrophils than eosinophils in their submucosa but a lack of inspissated secretions. Interestingly, if these patients are resuscitated, they have a rapid recovery.

Pathophysiology of "Steroid-Resistant" Asthma

Almost 30 years ago it was recognized that certain severe asthmatic patients do not respond appropriately to corticosteroids. These patients have become labeled as "steroid-resistant" or "steroid-insensitive." This condition is rarely reported but is perhaps underrecognized. In order to diagnose a "steroid-resistant" asthmatic (SRA), one needs first to establish that the patient does indeed have asthma and not another cause of wheezing, such as fixed airway obstruction, vocal cord dysfunction, panic attacks, or COPD. In addition, the physician must also establish that the patient's asthma has been maximally treated. For example, patient adherence, technique of inhaler use, and removal of offending agents in the individual's environment (e.g., family pets, cockroaches, dust mites) should be addressed. Furthermore, the physician needs to address other medical factors that can exacerbate the patient's asthma, including GERD, rhinitis, and sinusitis. Traditionally, if these conditions are met and maintained strictly for at least 6 months, it is possible to diagnose a patient as "steroid-resistant."

The exact mechanisms of steroid resistance have not been defined, but current work suggests two possibilities. Corticosteroids (GC) typically bind to the glucocorticoid receptor (GCR) and are then translocated to the nucleus. In the nucleus, this complex either interferes with or up-regulates certain genes that control cytokine and growth factor production. The GCR-GC complex requires interaction with transcription factors such as AP-1 and

NF-κB to complete this step. Therefore two distinct mechanisms for steroid resistance have been proposed. One mechanism centers on abnormal activation of the transcription factors. The other mechanism centers on the abnormalities of the GCR, including decreased numbers, decreased affinity between the GC and GCR, and decreased affinity between the GCR and the target gene. Some work has suggested defects on some of the receptors on peripheral blood mononuclear cells, whereas other studies suggest that there is a greater degree of activation of the CD4+ and CD8+ cells in these patients.

Summary

Bronchial asthma is a common debilitating condition that typically presents in childhood and will persist through adulthood in many of these patients. Typical symptoms include cough, chest tightness, wheezing, and shortness of breath that are secondary to reversible bronchoconstriction. Advances in the study of respiratory disease and allergy have demonstrated that inflammation of the airways is central to producing this hyperresponsiveness and bronchoconstriction. In addition, airway inflammation may also produce changes in the respiratory parenchyma and eventually lead to permanent airway obstruction.

The exact trigger causing the recruitment of inflammatory cells, notably the mast cell, eosinophil, and CD4+ T lymphocyte, is not completely understood. Currently, it is thought that many factors, both genetic and environmental, play a role in the appearance and persistence of airway inflammation in asthma. Furthermore, many of the environmental changes that play a role in the etiology and pathogenesis of asthma are directly linked to the Westernization of society, and therefore may explain the increasing prevalence, mortality, and morbidity of asthma.

▓   ▓   ▓

Key Points

- Asthma prevalence more than doubled in the last part of the 20th century, most likely due to changes in the environment and technological advances associated with the Westernization of society.
- Eighty percent of diagnoses of asthma are made by 6 years of age.
- In most patients (>80%), asthma persists into adulthood. The severity of childhood asthma appears to determine the likelihood of asthma in adulthood.
- The onset of asthma most likely arises from an interaction between genetic and environmental influences. Environmental influences include exposure to triggers of the disease, such as allergens, respiratory infections,

tobacco smoke, and pollution. It has also been hypothesized that protection from exposure to infections during early childhood may cause a predisposition to asthma by affecting the development of the immune system.

- The pathogenesis of asthma involves several different inflammatory cells (e.g., mast cells, T lymphocytes, B lymphocytes, eosinophils, basophils, neturophils) and mediators (e.g., histamine, leukotrienes, prostaglandins, interleukins).

- Chronic inflammation leads to remodeling of the airways, fixed changes in the airway resulting in nonreversible obstruction.

■   ■   ■

REFERENCES

1. **Weiss KB, Sullivan SD, Lyttle CS.** Trends in the cost of illness for asthma in the United States, 1985-1994. J Allergy Clin Immunol. 2000;106:493–9.

2. **Adams PF, Marano MA.** Current estimates from the National Health Interview Survey, 1994, Series 10: Data from the National Health Survey.

3. **Klebba AJ, Scott JH.** Estimates of selected comparability ratios based on dual coding of 1976 death certificates by the eighth and ninth revisions of the International Classification of Diseases. DHEW Publication (PHS) 80-112-28 (supplement), 1980.

4. **Martinez FD, Wright AL, Taussig LM, et al.** Asthma and wheezing in the first six years of life. N Engl J Med. 1995;332:133–8.

5. **Roorda RJ, Geritsen J, van Aalderen WMC, et al.** Follow-up of asthma from childhood to adulthood: influence of potential childhood risk factors on the outcome of pulmonary function and bronchial responsiveness in adulthood. J Allergy Clin Immunol. 1994;93:575–84.

6. **Strachan DP.** Hay fever, hygiene, and household size. BMJ. 1989;299:1259–60.

7. **Shaheen SO, Aaby P, Hall AJ, et al.** Measles and atopy in Guinea-Bissau. Lancet. 1996;347:1792–6.

8. **Matricardi PM, Rosmini F, Ferrigno L, et al.** Cross-sectional retrospective study of prevalence of atopy among Italian military students with antibodies against hepatitis A virus. BMJ. 1997;314:999–1003.

9. **Shirakawa T, Enomoto T, Shimazu S, Hopkin JM.** The inverse association between tuberculin responses and atopic disorder. Science. 1997;275:77–9.

10. **von Hertzen L, Klaukka T, Mattila H, Haahtela T.** *Mycobacterium tuberculosis* infection and the subsequent development of asthma and allergic conditions. J Allergy Clin Immunol. 1999;104:1211-4.

11. **Paunio M, Heinonen OP, Virtanen M, et al.** Measles history and atopic diseases: a population-based cross-sectional study. JAMA. 2000;283:343–6.

12. **Keeley DJ, Neill P, Gallivan S.** Comparison of the prevalence in reversible airways obstruction in rural and urban Zimbabwean children. Thorax. 1991;46:549–3.

13. **Saarinen UM, Karjosaari M.** Breastfeeding as prophylaxis against atopic disease: prospective follow-up study until 17 years old. Lancet. 1995;346:1065–9.

2

General Approach to the Evaluation and Management of an Adult with Asthma

Robert E. Reisman, MD
Raymond G. Slavin, MD

The diagnosis *asthma* does not in itself define its frequency or severity. Asthma may range from very mild symptoms limited to exercise or excessive pollen exposure (Case 2-1), to chronic daily wheeze, cough, and dyspnea. The appropriate evaluation and treatment is generally geared to the extent of individual reactions. For example, allergy evaluation is an important aspect of assessment of chronic asthma but may be unnecessary for the adolescent whose asthma is confined to strenuous exercise. National Heart, Lung and Blood Institute (NHLBI) therapeutic guidelines for treatment of asthma of differing degrees and severity have been developed and are widely applied. This chapter addresses the general concepts of the overall approach to evaluation and management of asthma; more detailed discussion of environmental control, pharmacotherapy, and immunotherapy can be found in Chapters 5, 6, and 7, respectively.

Goals of Therapy

The goals of asthma therapy are to minimize symptoms, prevent acute exacerbations and hospitalizations, normalize lung function as much as possible, and prevent the development of progression to a chronic asthmatic process with permanent lung damage (remodeling). With successful therapy these goals should be achieved with little or no adverse side effects.

CASE 2-1   *Asthma associated with severe seasonal allergic rhinitis*

A 20-year-old male with acute symptoms of allergic rhinitis is seen in late August. He has had fairly typical symptoms of nasal congestion with associated sneezing, itching, and rhinorrhea. He reports mild wheezing for the past few days, which has occurred previously, usually associated with severe nasal symptoms, at the same time of year. He is well the rest of the year and has had asthma on several other occasions only when in contact with cats. On physical examination, his nasal membranes appear swollen and pale, partially obstructing the nasal passages. There is mild expiratory wheezing with forced expiration. His peak expiratory flow is 400, about 75% predicted.

Discussion

This patient requires treatment for allergic rhinitis, which should also indirectly help to diminish asthma. The treatment for his rhinitis, in view of severity, should include the use of oral steroids for a short period of time, intranasal steroids, and perhaps combination antihistamine-decongestants. Specific treatment for his asthma probably can be confined to the use of an aerosol bronchodilator.

Symptom assessment reflecting asthma severity can easily be evaluated by asking the patient three questions:

1. Do you awaken at night with respiratory symptoms such as cough, wheezing, and shortness of breath?
2. Are your usual or normal activities modified because of breathing problems?
3. Do you have symptoms on awakening in the morning?

People with adequately controlled asthma should sleep throughout the night (relative to asthma), have no limitation of normal activities, and not awaken with morning respiratory symptoms. When asthma begins to deteriorate, these are early symptoms that dictate more aggressive therapy.

Normalization of lung function is an important goal of therapy. Periodic spirometry and frequent home measurements of peak expiratory flow rates can be important parameters of asthma control assessment. The peak flow measurement is particularly helpful for monitoring a subgroup of asthmatics who have difficulty perceiving subjective signs of increasing asthma. It also provides an objective assessment of asthma variability and medication effectiveness.

In the past, it was thought that in the absence of cigarette smoke exposure asthma rarely, if ever, led to chronic lung changes and irreversible disease. It is now apparent that persistent asthma can lead to chronic disease and fibrosis or scarring of lung tissue ("remodeling"). Thus an important goal of asthma management is to start treatment early and appropriately to prevent progression to irreversible disease.

Approaches to Management

There are two approaches for optimal asthma management: 1) identification and elimination or control of asthma triggers, and 2) medication designed for immediate relief and long-term control. Both of these aspects of management must be individualized.

Asthma Triggers

Single or multiple triggers may be responsible for inciting each individual's asthmatic reaction (Table 2-1). These are discussed below.

Allergy

Inhalant allergy is a common trigger of asthma. Potential allergens include nonseasonal or perennial inhalants (e.g., dust mites, cockroaches, and animal danders, particularly cats, dogs, horses, and small animals such as guinea pigs and gerbils) and seasonal inhalants (e.g., mold and pollen). All persons with asthma should be evaluated for the possibility of a contributory allergic etiology. The need for testing for contributory inhalant allergy may in some cases be based on the history—for example, in patients with only exercise-induced asthma, allergy evaluation may not be necessary—but some testing is generally required. Given the importance of allergens and their control to asthma morbidity and asthma management, the NHLBI Expert Panel recommended that patients with persistent asthma who require daily therapy be particularly evaluated for allergens as possible contributory factors.

The skin test is the allergy test of choice. It is sensitive, the results are immediately available, and cost is minimal. When skin testing is not possible (e.g., lack of trained personnel for testing, presence of extensive skin disease, concomitant use of antihistamines), serum analysis (RAST) in a reputable laboratory is reasonable.

The diagnosis of clinical allergy is dependent upon detection of allergen specific IgE and correlation of symptoms with exposure. This leads to environmental control measures and allergen immunotherapy, both discussed in detail in Chapters 5 and 7.

Avoidance of triggers that cause asthma is first-line treatment (see Chapter 5). Useful guidelines for minimizing dust mite exposure include

---

Table 2-1   Potential "Triggers" of Asthma

• Allergy	• Psychological factors
• Infection	• Medication
• Exercise	• Associated medical problems
• Airborne irritants	

removal of carpeting, obtaining covers for the pillow, box springs, and mattress, and adequate washing of bedding. Animal avoidance may be essential. Unfortunately, attempts to minimize exposure, such as keeping animals out of the bedroom and regular washing of animals, frequently is not adequate. In addition to the more common cat and dog exposure, small animals such as guinea pigs can be potent triggers of asthma.

Unless the history is clear-cut, recommending animal avoidance without confirmatory allergy testing is unreasonable and may be inappropriate. Likewise, environmental control of dust mite exposure, which does entail considerable effort and expense, should only be recommended if allergy is verified. Seasonal inhalant exposure can be minimized by keeping windows closed in the home and car and using air conditioning.

Most studies conclude that allergen immunotherapy, if given in adequate doses with appropriate allergens, is effective treatment for allergy-induced asthma. Clinical efficacy has often been correlated with decreased allergen-induced bronchial reactivity. Well-studied allergens for immunotherapy include tree, grass, and ragweed pollens, dust mites, dogs, cats, and, to a lesser extent, mold. Because asthma has a multifactorial etiology, the clinical evaluation of immunotherapy can be difficult. However, for many people with asthma, immunotherapy leads to decreased symptoms and less medication and potentially shortens the natural history of the disease process. Reassessment of the effectiveness of immunotherapy should be done after 2 or 3 years of treatment.

Infection

Upper respiratory infections, usually viral, are a very common cause of asthma exacerbations and probably the major reason for emergency room visits, urgent care, and hospitalization. Early treatment with more potent asthma medications (e.g., oral steroids) is essential. Although most of these infections are viral, antibiotics are frequently prescribed, particularly if sinusitis is suspected. All persons with asthma should receive yearly flu immunization (unless allergic to egg) and appropriate Pneumovax immunization.

Exercise

Almost all persons with asthma will develop symptoms with exercise. The exercise-induced asthmatic reaction (EIA) is dependent primarily upon the intensity of exercise, the environmental temperature, and the baseline lung function before exercise. Guidelines for medication prophylaxis and warm-up exercises usually lead to control and allow asthmatics to exercise and even compete competitively.

Recognition of the diagnosis of exercise-induced asthma is obviously important in order to utilize appropriate therapy. We have been impressed with the large number of people who complain of exercise-related shortness of breath or cough as the primary symptoms and are either diagnosed as "being out of shape" or treated with antihistamines or cough suppressants.

Problems have often persisted for several years before the basic diagnosis of exercise-induced asthma is made and proper therapy prescribed. Further discussion of EIA can be found in Chapter 8.

Irritants

Airborne irritants (e.g., fumes, strong odors, smoke, cold air) are common triggers of asthma. A common analogy is to consider the asthmatic bronchial membrane as "an open sore"; thus reactions are triggered following exposure to a variety of potential irritants. Cigarette smoke is particularly harmful and an almost universal asthma trigger. One renowned allergist commenting on this issue has cautioned other physicians, "If you treat a patient with asthma while that patient continues to smoke, you are helping that patient towards death."

Cold-air exposure is another almost universal trigger. Simple measures, such as wearing a scarf over the mouth to reduce cold exposure, can be very helpful. Individuals vary in their responses to other potential irritants such as perfume, paint, and chemical fumes. Weather and weather changes may be more subtle and less tangible irritants provoking asthma. Smog, high humidity, and cold damp air are often associated with asthma exacerbations. Temperature and barometric pressure changes are less obvious factors.

Psychological Factors/Stress

Opinions vary on the role of stress or emotional factors as an etiology for asthma exacerbations. These opinions range from viewing asthma as primarily an emotional disease to rejecting any relationship between psychological factors and asthma. Our opinion reflects a middle ground. Although not the prime cause of asthma, for some patients stress is an important trigger. That possibility should be evaluated in people with recurrent or chronic disease. Recognition of this relationship and, when needed, appropriate counseling and/or medication can be important therapy leading to decreased asthma symptoms.

Medications

Aspirin and other nonsteroidal anti-inflammatory drugs may cause acute asthma exacerbations, usually in people with a background of nasal polyps and sinusitis (see Chapter 13). This association is usually self-evident, although patients must be educated regarding potential dangers of all nonsteroidal anti-inflammatory drugs and hidden sources of aspirin such as Alka Seltzer.

Beta-blockers (e.g., Propranolol) accentuate asthma and are contraindicated unless absolutely necessary. Any asthmatic reaction is likely to be worse in the presence of beta-blocker therapy.

Associated Medical Problems

Associated medical problems may initiate and aggravate asthma. These include chronic sinusitis, GE reflux, and cardiac disease. These possibilities should be considered in the history and physical examination evaluation. Common symptoms suggestive of chronic sinus disease are postnasal drainage, daily cough, purulent secretions, and perhaps nasal congestion and headache. Gastroesophageal reflux should be suspected when patients complain of recurrent heartburn, belching, or upper abdominal distress. The presence of concomitant cardiac failure may initiate wheezing; this was formerly referred to as *cardiac asthma*. Treatment must be directed at cardiac factors in addition to bronchial reactivity.

Pharmacotherapy

Asthma medications can be divided into two therapeutic groups: 1) those designed for immediate symptom relief (quick-relief medications), such as inhaled albuterol, and 2) those designed to minimize inflammation and hopefully prevent chronic changes of remodeling (long-term control medication).

The appropriate evaluation of and subsequent therapeutic recommendations for each patient are very much dependent upon previous medication experience and response. The concepts of medical treatment discussed in detail in Chapter 6 are threefold:

1. Medication, usually inhaled albuterol, for immediate relief of acute symptoms.
2. Anti-inflammatory medication, usually inhaled steroids, for long-term "healing."
3. Medication, usually oral or injectable steroids, for early treatment of asthma exacerbations.

Guidelines for asthma management, based upon the degree and severity of symptoms, have been developed by a National Institute of Health Expert Panel. These concepts provide a very useful tool for optimal asthma management and disease control. Asthma is divided into four categories: mild intermittent, mild persistent, moderate persistent, and severe persistent. Medication requirements are based upon this classification.

- *Mild intermittent asthma* is defined as occasional exacerbations requiring the use of a short-acting bronchodilator less than twice a week. No daily controller medication is needed. Nocturnal symptoms occur less than twice a month. The one-second forced expiratory volume (FEV_1) or peak expiratory flow (PEF) is greater than 80% predicted.
- *Mild persistent asthma* requires more frequent use of short-acting bronchodilators. Daily controller medication, preferably inhaled steroids, is recommended. Symptoms occur more than two times a week but not more than once daily. Activity may be affected. Nocturnal symptoms are more than two times a month. The FEV_1 or PEF is greater than 80% predicted.
- *Moderate persistent asthma* is defined as daily symptoms not controlled by low-dose inhaled steroids (Case 2-2). Therapeutic recommendations

---

CASE 2-2   *Moderate persistent asthma*

A 32-year-old male presents with a 3-year history of asthma. He reports that the asthma occurs daily and he is awakened at night 2 or 3 times a week. Physical activities are frequently limited because of his asthma. He does have some concomitant nasal congestion. He is not aware of any obvious trigger for his asthma.

Pertinent physical examination findings are swollen nasal turbinates with a patent nasal airway, normal-appearing posterior pharynx, and generalized expiratory wheezing. His FEV_1 is 60% predicted and increased to 75% predicted after bronchodilators.

Discussion

This individual with moderate persistent asthma needs evaluation regarding possible triggers for asthma and certainly needs more medication. Detailed history should include potential exposure to allergens (e.g., pollen, mold, dust mite, animal danders), exposure to irritants such as cigarette smoke, and presence of symptoms suggestive of associated medical problems such as sinusitis or GE reflux. Allergy testing is most important because an allergic basis for this patient's asthma (and rhinitis) is highly suspect.

Immediate medication adjustment to control asthma should include higher doses of a more potent inhaled steroid (e.g., fluticasone, budesonide) and perhaps a long-acting bronchodilator.

---

include higher dose inhaled steroids and addition of long-acting beta-agonists. We would also recommend use of the newer more potent inhaled steroids such as fluticasone or budesonide. Additional considerations are the use of leukotriene modifiers and theophylline. In this category nocturnal symptoms occur more than once weekly. The FEV_1 or PEF is between 60% and 80% predicted, with PEF variability of greater than 30%.

• *Severe persistent asthma* is defined as continuous symptoms interfering with sleep and physical activity *and* frequent exacerbations, despite the use of the aforementioned medications. Oral steroids are usually required. Very high doses of inhaled steroids, particularly the more potent inhaled steroids, also may be prescribed. Lung function is less than 60% predicted, and PEF variability is greater than 30%.

Because degrees of asthma may change from one category to another, medication requirements need to be adjusted. The overall purpose is to provide minimum medication that ensures the goals of symptom control and maximal lung function.

Cost is another factor that often needs consideration. The more effective preferable asthma medications, such as inhaled steroids and leukotriene modifiers, are relatively expensive. Affordability and thus compliance with drug usage as prescribed may be an issue for such patients as those on Medicare without prescription drug coverage. Provision of drug samples and substitution of less expensive therapeutically effective medication are often extremely important aspects of successful therapy.

Individual Patient Assessment

The application of the concepts of asthma management—recognition and control of triggers and appropriate medication—must be individualized for each person with asthma. The basis for this individual assessment depends on a number of factors: history of frequency and severity of asthma, recognition of triggering factors, medication experience, other associated allergic and health issues, physical examination findings, and lung function assessment.

History

The details of asthma frequency (daily, perennial, seasonal, nocturnal, time of day) and environmental relationship (home, work, indoors, outdoors) will help establish potential etiologies or triggers. The simple question "What makes your asthma worse and what makes it better?" is extremely helpful.

Commonly requested information that may be useful in identifying allergic triggers includes animal exposure, feather (pillows) exposure, types of heating (hot air tends to increase dust exposure), potential dust mite collectors particularly in the bedroom (e.g., carpeting, furniture, mattresses), and potential mold exposure (e.g., damp areas, basements). Seasonal frequency suggests pollen or outdoor mold allergy. Early morning and evening worsening may be related to pollen exposure, which is greater at that time. Potential irritant exposures are certainly cigarette smoke, excessive amounts of dust or mold, and temperature and humidity extremes. Potential allergens or irritants in the work environment need to be explored if asthma exacerbates with that exposure.

Medication experience is extremely useful in recognizing asthma severity and dictating future medical advice. For example, if inhaled beclomethasone in reasonable dose has not adequately controlled asthma, other types of medication should be prescribed, such as more potent inhaled steroids. The occurrence of acute exacerbations of asthma requiring emergency care or hospitalization is a prediction of potential asthma severity and more urgent need for appropriate management. In this regard, details of the symptoms leading up to the emergency treatment may provide insight into early therapy in the future, which could abort more serious symptoms. For example, the early use of prednisone at the first sign of an upper airway infection may prevent progression to serious asthma.

The presence of allergic upper airway disease, such as seasonal rhinitis, suggests that allergic triggers may be important aspects of asthma. A family history of allergic disease also suggests potential personal allergy. However, while interesting, clinical decision making regarding allergy evaluation is not made based on the presence or lack of presence of family members with allergic problems.

As mentioned, associated health issues such as chronic sinusitis, GE reflux, and cardiac failure may directly affect asthma. In addition, medications prescribed for other reasons, such as beta-blockers, may aggravate asthma.

It is important to appreciate that asthma is a clinical spectrum. At one end is the patient who complains of wheezing and shortness of breath. At the other end is the patient who only coughs. Coughing with exercise or at night may mean asthma, although there is no associated wheezing or breathlessness. The etiology and treatment of "cough variant asthma" should be approached in the same fashion as more typical asthma.

Physical Examination

Physical examination may be entirely normal, particularly if patients are asymptomatic at that time. The classic sign of asthma is expiratory wheezing. Severe asthma is associated with increased respiratory rate and sternomastoid muscle retraction.

There are helpful physical examination findings: lack of chest expansion with inspiration, suggesting significant chronic obstructive pulmonary disease; nasal polyps, suggesting asthma as having a specific pattern (aspirin triad or Samter's triad); pale swollen nasal membranes, suggesting an allergic problem; and purulent secretions or a "cobblestone" appearance of the posterior pharynx, suggesting sinusitis.

Lung Function Tests

All patients who have recurrent or perennial asthma should have lung function evaluation. This is an important aspect of assessment of asthma severity and monitoring disease. Diagnosing or managing asthma without pulmonary function testing is like trying to control hypertension without blood pressure readings. Abnormal or deteriorating lung function suggests inadequate asthma control and dictates more intensive medical therapy and perhaps better control of pertinent triggers. Spirometry should be done about once a year. At the initial visit, demonstrating reversibility of airway obstruction with an inhaled bronchodilator such as albuterol is helpful in making a diagnosis of asthma. This is defined as a 15% to 20% increase in FEV_1. Spirometry is particularly helpful if done when a patient is relatively asymptomatic. If abnormal in that situation, additional therapy would be indicated, despite the patient's lack of symptoms.

PEF measurements, recorded at the time of each office visit and, for many people, at home on a daily basis, may provide a helpful ongoing assessment. Patients must be instructed in the proper technique for using the peak flow meter to ensure accuracy of recordings. For some patients, an objective number, which reflects the degree of asthma, is a very helpful parameter for understanding their disease, its triggers, and the effect of medication. Based upon PEF, asthma action plans have been developed and these can be very helpful. If the PEF decreases from its usual personal best by 25%, an increase in medication may be indicated. If the PEF decreases by 50%, an office visit is necessary for further treatment such as oral steroids.

Allergy Tests

As mentioned previously, an allergy etiology should be considered for patients with asthma. Allergy is generally a more likely etiology in patients whose asthma starts before the age of 35 to 40, but it can be important even in elderly people. Inhalant allergens (e.g., pollen, dust, mold, animal danders) are the major problems.

Food allergy is a rare cause for asthma not associated with generalized allergic symptoms, such as urticaria, angioedema, and hypotension. Food allergy tests are usually not needed as part of routine evaluation.

The specifics of allergy tests are dependent upon historical details of asthma frequency and relationship to possible allergic triggers. In addition to obvious allergen-induced asthma (e.g., cat exposure), details of home and occupational environment may provide important information.

Most people with perennial or recurrent symptoms should be tested with both indoor and outdoor allergens (e.g., pollen, dust mite, mold). Cockroach allergy can be an important issue, particularly for inner-city residents with asthma. People with asthma that is confined to certain times of the year or specific exposure can usually be adequately evaluated with fewer tests.

Other Tests

Chest x-rays are generally normal and rarely helpful unless complicating pneumonia or lung conditions are suspected. A baseline chest x-ray is generally recommended if asthma is a frequent or chronic problem.

Sinus CT scans are indicated if chronic sinus disease is suspected, a potential major trigger for asthma.

Management Skills

Inhaled medication is now the prime mode of asthma therapy. Appropriate use of an inhaler is obviously necessary to ensure adequate delivery of medication to the lower airways. Patients should be instructed in the proper use of an inhaler and the technique reviewed regularly. Spacers are often useful adjuncts that assure proper deposition of inhaled medication. Eventually, all aerosolized medication will be replaced by breath-actuated powdered-dose devices.

As mentioned earlier, peak expiratory flow meters used at home to monitor lung function are extremely helpful.

Monitoring

For people who have recurrent or chronic symptoms, monitoring of asthma is essential. Basically, there are two parameters to be considered: symptoms and lung function. Symptoms are assessed by questions about nocturnal awakening, limitation of exercise function, and need for reliever medication. Measurement of peak flows can be very helpful and are particularly important for a subset of people who have poor perception of clinical deterioration.

Early treatment of exacerbations is important to limit symptoms and prevent hospitalization. We encourage patient communication with the physician for advice at the earliest sign of symptom exacerbation or decreased lung function. Although allergy treatment plans have been suggested and are useful, physician contact is still preferable at the time of any exacerbation of symptoms.

Periodic reassessment of asthma is important and should be contingent upon the frequency and severity of asthma. People who need daily mediation for control should be seen on a regular basis, perhaps every 1 to 2 months for this reassessment. Patients with less severe problems may be seen less frequently. The NHLBI guidelines suggest pulmonary function tests every 1 to 2 years.

Patient Education

People with asthma should be well educated regarding the disease process, triggers, ongoing assessment of disease activity, and benefits and side effects of medication. Numerous avenues for education are available, including personal physician and health care provider discussion, group sessions sponsored by organizations such as the American Academy of Allergy, Asthma, and Immunology; American College of Allergy, Asthma and Immunology; the Asthma and Allergy Foundation of America; and the American Lung Association. These organizations provide excellent written material and video presentations.

Key Points

- The goals of asthma therapy are to minimize symptoms, prevent acute exacerbations and hospitalization, normalize lung function as much as possible, and prevent chronic disease that can lead to airway remodeling.

- One aspect of asthma management is identification and elimination or control of asthma triggers (e.g., allergens, infection, exercise, irritants, medications, associated medical problems).

- Pharmacotherapy for asthma consists of medications for symptom relief and for long-term control of inflammation and prevention of airway remodeling.

- Asthma is divided into four categories: 1) mild intermittent, 2) mild persistent, 3) moderate persistent, and 4) severe persistent.

- Asthma management must be individualized based on the history of asthma severity and frequency, triggers, other allergy and health problems, physical examination findings, and lung function assessment.

■   ■   ■

SUGGESTED READING

Abramson MJ, Puy RM, Weiner JM. Is allergen immunotherapy effective in asthma? A meta-analysis of randomized controlled trials. Am J Respir Crit Care Med. 1995;151: 969–74.

Barnes PJ. Current issues for establishing inhaled corticosteroids as the anti-inflammatory agents of choice in asthma. J Allergy Clin Immunol. 1998;101:S427–33.

Gibson PG. Monitoring the patient with asthma: an evidence-based approach. J Allergy Clin Immunol. 2000;106:17–26.

Li JTC. Do peak flow meters lead to better asthma control? J Res Dis. 1995;16:381–98.

National Heart, Lung and Blood Institute. Highlights of the Expert Panel Report 2: Guidelines for the Diagnosis and Management of Asthma. Bethesda, MD: National Institute of Health, 1997; NIH Publication 97-40051A.

Platts-Mills TAE, Vaughan JW, Carter MC, Woodfolk JA. The role of intervention in established allergy: avoidance of indoor allergies in the treatment of chronic allergic disease. J Allergy Clin Immunol. 2000;106:787–804.

3

■ ■ ■

Differential Diagnosis of Asthma

Tammy Heinly, MD

Phillip L. Lieberman, MD

Asthma affects approximately 15 million Americans. It is a progressive disease of the airways that is marked by bronchial hyperactivity, mucous production, and cellular infiltration causing airway wall edema. This inflammatory component is progressive and may be irreversible if not properly diagnosed and treated. Cough, wheeze, and dyspnea are common asthma symptoms. These symptoms, however, may also occur with other disorders that are often misdiagnosed as asthma. Thus one must be aware of the differential diagnosis (Tables 3-1 and 3-2) of this common condition (1-4).

Chronic Obstructive Pulmonary Disease

The most frequent clinical entities to be considered in the differential diagnoses of asthma are *chronic obstructive pulmonary disease* (COPD) disorders—namely, chronic bronchitis and emphysema. *Chronic bronchitis* is diagnosed clinically by the presence of a chronic productive cough for three months in each of two successive years during which no other cause can be identified. *Emphysema* is characterized by abnormal permanent enlargement of the air spaces distal to the terminal bronchioles accompanied by destruction of their walls without obvious fibrosis, although recent evidence indicates that subtle fibrotic changes can occur. In both chronic bronchitis and emphysema, there is marked inflammation, but in both diseases it is distinct from the unique form of eosinophilic inflammation characteristic of asthma.

Asthma is characterized by eosinophilic airway inflammation, airway hyperresponsiveness, and reversible air flow obstruction. However, it is

Table 3-1   Differential Diagnosis of Asthma in Adults

Obstructive Lung Disease
Chronic bronchitis
Emphysema

Mechanical Obstruction
Vocal cord paralysis
Glottic web
Posttraumatic injury (surgical,
   endotracheal tube)
 Laryngeal stenosis
 Subglottic stenosis
Laryngotracheomalacia with
   relapsing polychondritis
Primary and secondary neoplasia
Foreign body

Cardiac Disorders
Cardiogenic venous hypertension
Mitral valve prolapse
Atrial myxoma

Somatoform Disorders
Vocal cord dysfunction
Hyperventilation syndrome

Systemic Disorders
Cystic fibrosis
Mastocytosis
Carcinoid

Table 3-2   Differential Diagnosis of Asthma in Children and Adolescents

- Cystic fibrosis

- Bronchopulmonary dysplasia

- Foreign body

- Gastroesophageal reflux

- Tracheoesophageal fistula

- Laryngeal web

- Congestive heart failure

- Bronchiolitis

- Pertussis

- Tuberculosis

- Congenital vascular ring

- Immune deficiency (recurrent
  pneumonia and bronchiectasis)

- Bronchiolitis obliterans

important to note that in some asthmatics, complete air flow reversibility cannot be achieved, a finding more traditionally considered to be consistent with emphysema and bronchitis.

It should also be noted that patients with chronic bronchitis may not exhibit airway obstruction and that some patients with emphysema and bronchitis do experience air flow reversibility. Finally, quite often COPD and asthma exist together. Therefore it is understandable that, although these conditions can be defined with reasonable precision, the application of the definitions clinically is often imprecise, and distinctions between these disorders blur. This is perhaps especially true regarding chronic bronchitis and asthma, thus prompting the hybrid term *asthmatic bronchitis*, a diagnosis with an established ICD code but one which "begs the question" nonetheless. Thus, in practice, clear-cut distinctions between these disorders sometimes are not possible, and empiric therapy must be initiated based on the "best possible educated guess."

Nevertheless, there are features of each disease that are very helpful in making diagnostic distinctions. Many factors may be helpful in distinguishing asthma from COPD, including pertinent historical and physical findings. The mean age at presentation of a patient with COPD is 64.6 years (4). This, in conjunction with a history of tobacco abuse and the lack of a family history of asthma, points more towards a diagnosis of COPD. Asthma is more likely to present much earlier (about 80% of asthmatics start by age 6), and a positive family history of asthma is often elicited. The physical examination of a patient with COPD may include the following abnormalities: wheezing, prolonged expiratory phase, barrel chest deformity, diminished chest expansion on inspiration, decreased subxiphoid apical impulse, and hyperresonance. These findings may fluctuate in severity but are always present to some extent. In contrast, the examination of the asthmatic patient may be normal or may include wheezing and a prolonged expiratory phase.

Although the history and physical examination may be helpful in distinguishing between COPD and asthma in most patients, spirometry and chest radiographs remain essential. Typically asthmatics have greater airway hyperreactivity and greater reversibility following the inhalation of beta-2 agonists. Radiographically these two disorders may appear the same, with pulmonary hyperinflation, peribronchial thickening, and increased lung lucency. With bronchoalveolar lavage elevations in airway eosinophils are far more common in asthma though also noted in COPD; eosinophil degranulation and elevated levels of eosinophil cationic protein, however, are seen only in asthma (5). Elevation of peripheral blood eosinophils is also characteristic of asthma and not normally seen in COPD.

Table 3-3 summarizes the distinctions between asthma and COPD.

Mechanical Obstruction

Although chronic obstructive lung diseases are the most common masqueraders of asthma, other forms of obstruction can also mimic this disorder. Obstructive diseases of the larynx and trachea may result in common asthma symptoms such as cough, wheeze, and breathlessness.

There are many causes of obstruction at the level of the larynx, with vocal cord paralysis being the most common. This may result from trauma during surgery or endotracheal intubation. Primary or secondary neoplasms of the lung, larynx, or thyroid may result in vocal cord paralysis. Paralysis can occur by fibrosis and laryngeal stenosis secondary to granulomatous diseases, such as Wegener's granulomatosis, tuberculosis, and sarcoidosis. Inflammatory disorders such as rheumatoid arthritis can lead to fixation of the cricoarytenoid joint and produce vocal cord paralysis.

Many disorders that affect the larynx can also cause tracheal obstruction or stenosis (Case 3-1). Other entities to consider include laryngotracheomalacia,

Table 3-3   Distinguishing Asthma from Chronic Obstructive Pulmonary Disease

	Asthma	*COPD*
Mean age at presentation	29.6 years	64.6 years
Family history	Often positive	Noncontributory
Role of smoking	Less significant	Highly significant
Chest examination	Normal, wheezing, prolonged expiratory phase	Wheezing, hyperresonance, barrel chest deformity, subxiphoid apical impulse
Airway hyperreactivity	+++	++
Reversibility post-beta-2 agonist	+++	++
Radiographic findings	Pulmonary hyperinflation, peribronchial cuffing, elevated lung lucency	Pulmonary hyperinflation, peribronchial cuffing, elevated interstitial markings
Inflammatory component	Elevated number of eosinophils, elevated eosinophil cationic protein	CD8+ lymphocytes, macrophages

---

CASE 3-1   *Tracheal stenosis*

A 66-year-old woman is scheduled for total knee replacement. She had undergone uneventful endotracheal intubation and general anesthesia on two previous occasions. She had a history of asthma for which she took three inhalers. Her history was unremarkable except for dyspnea on exertion. Her most recent pulmonary function tests were FEV_1, 2.11 L (118%); FVC, 2.31 L (106%); and PEFR, 6.83 L/min (128%).

Diffuse wheezing was present during her preoperative physical examination. Chest radiography revealed significant tracheal narrowing, maximum at the level of thoracic vertebra 2, with a midline shift to the right (Fig. 3-1). On review of chest radiographs taken 5 years earlier, tracheal stenosis was evident. The patient was diagnosed with a fixed extrathoracic obstruction and was referred for appropriate surgery.

This case demonstrates that not all that wheezes is asthma.

---

which may be associated with relapsing polychondritis, and anatomic abnormalities such as tracheal web and vascular rings.

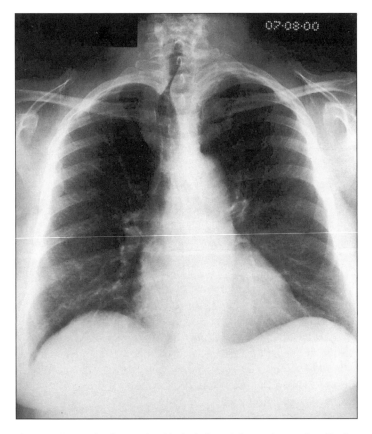

Figure 3-1   Tracheal stenosis with deviation of the trachea as described in Case 3-1.

Cardiac Disorders

Chest tightness, dyspnea on exertion, and breathlessness are common symptoms of both asthma and congestive heart failure. A thorough cardiovascular examination is essential in differentiating between these disorders. Careful attention should be paid to auscultation of murmurs and third heart sounds. Mitral valve prolapse and atrial septal defects may present with these chronic symptoms and may be diagnosed on the basis of physical examination alone.

Mitral valve disease may result in left-sided cardiac decompensation, which may mimic asthma. Cardiac asthma is due to airway vascular mechanisms (6). Vascular changes in the airway include engorgement of the microcirculation and an increase in intravascular hydrostatic pressure, leading to perivascular edema. This form of asthma responds best to diuretics and the inhalation of alpha-adrenergic vasoconstrictors. Partial response may also be observed with the use of beta-2 agonists as there is an associated increase in bronchial hyperreactivity. It is for this reason that for those patients who do not respond as expected to standard asthma therapy, left ventricular failure must also be considered. Right ventricular decompensation may also present with acute shortness of breath and dyspnea on exertion as seen with pulmonary emboli. This may mimic status asthmaticus in the emergency room setting. Differentiating features can include chest pain, hemoptysis, and an elevated A-a gradient.

Somatoform Disorders

Somatoform disorders such as hyperventilation and vocal cord dysfunction syndrome can present dramatically or as causes of chronic dyspnea. In either case they can mimic asthma.

Hyperventilation Disorders

Hyperventilation is defined as breathing in excess of metabolic requirements that is associated with increased carbon dioxide requirements (7). This can cause a variety of symptoms such as dyspnea, paresthesia, tingling of fingertips, confusion, dizziness, and palpitations. Hyperventilation was previously diagnosed by history alone, but today physical and emotional provocation tests can be employed. An example of a *physical provocation test* is the hyperventilation provocation test (HVPT). In this test patients are asked to voluntarily hyperventilate and the end-tidal pCO_2 (PET) is measured. Elevations in PET pCO_2 are correlated with the symptoms patients experience during the test. The word color conflict test (WCCT), an example of an *emotional provocation test*, can be used to determine if mental stress is triggering hyperventilation and associated symptoms.

These tests were recently validated in a study by Ringsberg et al (7). Ten patients with "asthma-like symptoms" were compared with ten known asthmatics and ten healthy controls. The patients underwent provocation by both physical and mental stimuli using HVPT and WCCT, respectively. The ten study subjects had a notably slower rate of recovery of end-tidal pCO_2 than the healthy controls following HVPT. In addition, more symptoms were reproduced in the subjects with "asthma-like symptoms" using WCCT. HVPT and WCCT may therefore be useful tools in establishing the diagnosis of hyperventilation.

Hyperventilation disorder has also been identified as the cause of exercise-induced symptoms in patients who respond poorly to beta-agonists. A recent study by Hammo et al evaluated 32 patients with a diagnosis of exercise-induced bronchospasm (8). The patients, who ranged in age from 8 to 18 years, underwent exercise challenge testing on a treadmill, and spirometry, oxygen saturation, and end-tidal pCO_2 were measured. Four of the 32 patients had a confirmed diagnosis of exercise-induced broncho-spasm with a decline in FEV_1 of greater than 15%. In 17 patients there were no spirometric changes and symptoms could not be reproduced. A diagnosis of hyperventilation syndrome was made in 11 patients who had a decline in FEV_1 of <15% and also experienced a decline in end-tidal pCO_2.

Patients with chronic dyspnea due to hyperventilation disorder often describe their symptoms in a characteristic fashion. The dyspnea is usually inspiratory in nature and is experienced as the inability to "get a deep-enough breath" or for the breath to "get to the bottom of the lungs". These patients also quite often exhibit "sighing respirations" during the interview and at the time of pulmonary function testing.

Vocal Cord Dysfunction

Vocal cord dysfunction is another example of a subconscious conversion disorder (9,10). Inappropriate adduction of the vocal cords during inspiration can cause symptoms that mimic asthma. Nocturnal symptoms are uncommon. As seen with asthma, stress, exercise, and irritant inhalants can trigger episodes. The overwhelming majority of the patients reported to date are young females, with a striking sex ratio of 9 females to 1 male. Vocal cord dysfunction has been reported in children and adolescents, especially those who strive for athletic or academic achievement (11). There is also a preponderance of health care workers with this disorder. The presentation of this disorder is often dramatic, leading to frequent emergency room visits and even mechanical ventilation.

Often these patients are diagnosed with asthma and inappropriately treated with oral and inhaled corticosteroids (Case 3-2). Prompt diagnosis limits the adverse effects of these medications. Diagnostic tools include physical examination, eosinophil count, pulmonary function testing, and rhinolaryngoscopy. The physical examination may be normal between episodes. During an exacerbation, clinical clues to this disorder include the ability to speak during an episode, wheezing or stridor that is more audible over the neck than lung fields, no hyperexpansion on chest radiograph, normal pCO_2 and A-a oxygen tension gradient, and no response to asthma medications. The flow volume loop is the crucial measurement of pulmonary function. Patients with vocal cord dysfunction experience slowing of inspiratory air flow that is disproportionate to their expiratory slowing. A flat inspiratory loop on flow volume testing is characteristic of vocal cord dysfunction (Fig. 3-2). Representative examples of spirometric abnormalities are shown in Figure 3-3. Rhinoscopy can be performed during an exacerbation. Inappropriate adduction of the vocal cords on inspiration can produce a characteristic "chink" deformity on laryngoscopic examination.

Treatment of vocal cord dysfunction involves a multidisciplinary approach. Speech therapy is essential to retrain the vocal cords to appropriately

---

CASE 3-2   *Vocal cord dysfunction*

A 35-year-old female hospital nurse presented for evaluation of asthma. Her illness had resulted in six hospitalizations and frequent emergency room visits (1 or 2 times per month). Her medical history was significant for common variable immunodeficiency, depression, and gastroesophageal reflux. Her medications included fluticasone 220 (Flovent) 2 puffs bid, salmeterol (Serevent) 2 puffs bid, montelukast sodium (Singulair) 10 mg daily, omeprazole (Prilosec), paroxetine HCl (Paxil), and intravenous immunoglobulin infusions. Despite this regimen she required oral steroid bursts on a monthly basis.

Her evaluation included negative allergy skin tests, normal sinus and chest radiographs, a total eosinophil count of 35 cell/mm^3, and spirometry as follows: FEV$_1$, 1.86 L (64%); FVC, 2.21 L (65%); and FEF 25–75, 2.05 L (61%). There was no reversibility after administration of albuterol.

Initially, she was placed on oral prednisone 40 mg daily for 10 days and her fluticasone 220 increased to 4 puffs bid. Her symptoms subsided within 24 hours, and 2 weeks later her repeat pulmonary functions had improved as follows: FEV$_1$, 2.51 L (87%); FVC, 2.93 L (86%); and FEF 25–75, 2.94 L (88%).

Three weeks afterwards, however, she returned to the office with complaints of cough, wheeze, and breathlessness. Her FEV$_1$ had decreased to 2.06 L (71% normal), improving to 2.21 L after albuterol nebulization. A flat inspiratory loop was noted (Fig. 3-2), and the patient underwent rhinolaryngoscopy in her physician's office. A chink deformity consistent with vocal cord dysfunction was noted, and the diagnosis of vocal cord dysfunction was made. The patient has undergone extensive speech therapy, counseling, and instruction on relaxation techniques.

As can be seen from this case, spirometry can be essential in establishing the correct diagnosis in cases of pulmonary disorders mimicking asthma.

---

abduct during inspiration. Psychotherapy may benefit relaxation techniques and underlying issues.

Systemic Disorders

We often only consider cystic fibrosis in the differential diagnosis of wheezing in infancy and early childhood. Yet more than one-third of all patients with cystic fibrosis are over 18 years old. In fact, over a 23-year period from 1969 to 1992 survival rates increased from 14 to 29.4 years (12). Therefore it is important that physicians familiarize themselves with this condition. Cystic fibrosis is the result of a three base pair deletion of phenylalanine. ΔF508 is the most common genetic mutation (12). Mutations of the cystic fibrosis transmembrane conductance regulator gene (CFTR) result in a block in the sodium and chloride transport at the epithelial level. This in turn

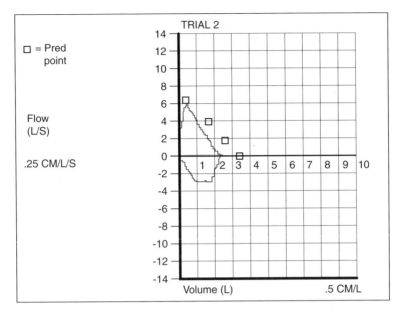

Figure 3-2 Flat inspiratory loop noted on spirometry consistent with a diagnosis of vocal cord dysfunction.

results in a decrease in sodium and water resorption at the mucosal surfaces of the respiratory and gastrointestinal tracts. Desiccation of airway epithelia leads to a more viscous mucus, thereby impairing mucociliary transport. This in turn leads to bronchial obstruction, pneumonias, and bronchiectasis. Cystic fibrosis is also marked by gastrointestinal malabsorption, pancreatic insufficiency, male infertility, and nonallergic nasal polyps.

Diagnosis of cystic fibrosis is confirmed by sweat test and subsequent DNA analysis. Treatment strategies include pharmacotherapy and gene therapy. In addition, cystic fibrosis has additional relevant associations to allergic disorders. Upper airway associations include nasal polyps and chronic sinusitis. Associated lower airway findings include allergic bronchopulmonary aspergillosis and increased bronchial hyperreactivity. In fact, cystic fibrosis is included in the list of disorders associated with a positive methacholine challenge test.

Mastocytosis and carcinoid are other systemic diseases that should be considered in the differential diagnosis of asthma. Both of these conditions can be associated with wheezing. However, there should be no difficulty in distinguishing them from asthma *per se*. In both instances cutaneous manifestations are present. In mastocytosis, flush, urticaria, and angioedema are found. In carcinoid, flushing is present. In addition, hypotension can occur during acute episodes of wheezing with mastocytosis. Thus it is rare for either of these two conditions to be confused with asthma.

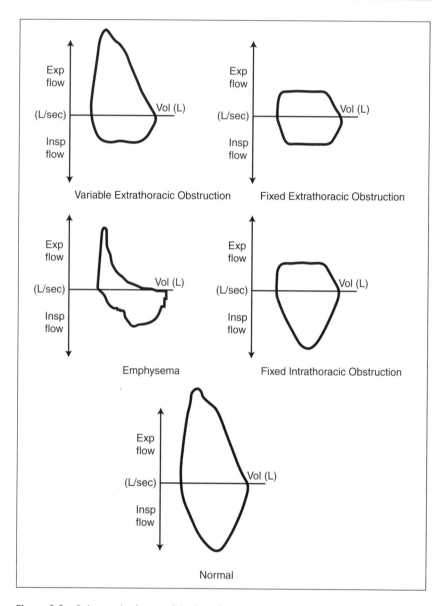

Figure 3-3   Spirometric abnormalities in pulmonary diseases mimicking asthma.

Related Pediatric Issues

An awareness of disorders that may mimic asthma in the pediatric population is important to physicians caring for adolescents and young adult patients. Anatomic abnormalities such as tracheoesophageal fistula, laryngeal web, and congenital vascular ring present early in childhood, whereas atrial septal defects may present as cardiac asthma in the second decade of life. Congenital or acquired immunodeficiencies may present with symptoms of asthma that are actually secondary to recurrent pneumonias or bronchiectasis. Again, mild forms of cystic fibrosis may also have a late presentation and be the cause of recurrent wheezing.

There are no specific diagnostic tools that alert the physician to these disorders; therefore a high degree of suspicion is essential. The diagnosis of pediatric conditions mimicking asthma depends upon ancillary tests such as chest x-ray, echocardiography, and the sweat test. In most instances the diagnosis is pursued when the response to standard therapy for asthma fails to control symptoms.

Conclusion

Because asthma symptoms such as cough, wheeze, and dyspnea also occur with other disorders, patients of all ages are often misdiagnosed with asthma. It is therefore imperative for physicians to be familiar with the differential diagnosis and to able to differentiate between asthma and the many disorders that may mimic this common condition.

Key Points

- Asthma symptoms such a cough, wheeze, and dyspnea are seen with other disorders, which are consequently misdiagnosed as asthma.
- The most important diseases to be considered in the differential diagnosis of asthma are chronic bronchitis and emphysema. Spirometry and chest radiography are essential in distinguishing these chronic obstructive pulmonary diseases (COPDs) from asthma.
- Because cardiac disorders such as mitral valve prolapse and congestive heart failure may present with symptoms of chest tightness, dyspnea on exertion, and breathlessness, a thorough cardiovascular examination may be essential in patients.
- The hyperventilation provocation test (HVPT) and word color conflict test (WCCT) can help establish the diagnosis of hyperventilation. Vocal cord dysfunction can be identified by flow volume loop abnormalities.
- Cystic fibrosis should be considered in the differential diagnosis of asthma for adults as well as for children.
- Differential diagnosis of asthma for children and adolescents should also be considered.

■   ■   ■

REFERENCES

1. **Milgrom H, Wood RP.** Respiratory conditions that mimic asthma. Immunology and Allergy Clinics of North America. 1998;18:113–32.

2. **Martinati LC, Boner AL.** Clinical diagnosis of wheezing in early childhood. Allergy. 1995;50:701–10.

3. **Flaherty KR, Kazerooni EA, Martinez FJ, et al.** Differential diagnosis of chronic airflow obstruction. J Asthma. 2000;37:201–23.

4. **Tilles SA, Nelson HS.** Differential diagnosis of adult asthma. Immunology and Allergy Clinics of North America. 1996;16:19–33.

5. **Jeffery PK.** Comparison of the structural and inflammatory features of COPD and asthma. Chest. 2000;117(suppl):251–60.

6. **Gilbert IA, McFadden ER Jr.** Vascular mechanisms in exercise induced asthma. In: Asthma and Rhinitis. Cambridge: Blackwell Science; 1995.

7. **Ringsberg KC, Akerlind I.** Presence of hyperventilation in patients with asthma-like symptoms but negative asthma test responses: provocation with voluntary hyperventilation and mental stress. J Allergy Clin Immunol. 1999;601–8.

8. **Hammo A, Weinberger MW.** Exercise-induced hyperventilation: a pseudo-asthma syndrome. Ann Allergy Asthma Immunol. 1999;82:574–8.

9. **Brugman SM, Newman K.** Vocal cord dysfunction. National Jewish Center for Immunology and Respiratory Medicine. Medical/Scientific Update. 1993;11:1–4.

10. **O'Hollaren MT.** Masqueraders in clinical allergy: laryngeal dysfunction causing dyspnea. Ann Allergy Asthma Immunol. 1990;65:351–6.

11. **Gavin LA, Wamboldt M, Brugman S, et al.** Psychological and family characteristics of adolescents with vocal cord dysfunction. J Asthma. 1998;35:409–17.

12. **Schwartz R.** Chronic pulmonary disease in children, including cystic fibrosis and primary dyskinesia. In: Bierman CW, Pearlman DS, Shapiro GG, eds. Allergy, Asthma, and Immunology from Infancy to Adulthood, 3rd ed. Philadelphia: WB Saunders; 1995.

4

Management of Acute Asthma in the Office Setting

Nina C. Ramirez, MD

Richard F. Lockey, MD

A sthma is the most treatable of all chronic diseases, and persons with asthma should rarely need emergency care or hospitalization. In spite of this, approximately 2 million people with asthma are treated in emergency rooms in the United States every year, 500,000 of whom require hospitalization because of the seriousness of their illness. In addition, approximately 5000 people die from asthma each year. The purposes of this chapter are

1. To identify the signs and symptoms of acute asthma.

2. To discuss the use of office-based physiologic and laboratory parameters in determining the severity of asthma.

3. To outline appropriate treatment strategies for patients presenting to an office or clinic with an acute, potentially life threatening, episode of asthma.

4. To provide the physician with criteria to determine when to hospitalize the patient with severe asthma.

5. To establish recommendations to help the patient avoid future severe episodes of asthma.

Goals of Asthma Therapy

The goals of asthma therapy, as outlined in *Guidelines for the Diagnosis and Management of Asthma* by the National Heart, Lung, and Blood Institute (1), are discussed in Chapter 2.

The physician treating a patient with asthma should be able to 1) recognize patients at greater risk for fatal asthma, 2) teach the patient to recognize the signs and symptoms of deteriorating asthma, 3) provide an action plan for the patient with asthma to initiate at the onset of an exacerbation, 4) be available to intercede if that action plan is not effective, and 5) identify and treat coexisting conditions, such as allergic rhinitis, sinusitis, gastroesophageal reflux, and obesity, which contribute to the morbidity and mortality associated with asthma.

Risk Factors for Near-Fatal and Fatal Asthma

Particular features in patient history have been associated with the risk for near-fatal and fatal asthma. These risk factors make the early recognition and treatment of an asthma exacerbation even more important.

Major risk factors for near-fatal and fatal asthma include a history of severe exacerbations requiring admission to an intensive care setting (especially an admission requiring intubation and mechanical ventilation), multiple emergency room visits and/or hospitalizations, and overuse of short-acting bronchodilators. Individuals who use a full container of a short-acting metered dose inhaler (MDI) beta-agonist every 2 weeks or even more frequently are at particular risk and may no longer appropriately respond to a beta-agonist because of subsensitivity. Other risk factors include the lack of recognition of the severity of airway obstruction by both the physician and/or the patient, recent withdrawal of a patient from systemic corticosteroids, and the failure of the physician to use anti-inflammatory drugs as primary therapy, particularly in patients with moderate-to-severe asthma. Other risk factors are psychiatric and socioeconomic problems and poor compliance by the patient and/or the family. Table 4-1 lists risk factors for near-fatal and fatal asthma (2).

Symptoms and Signs of Severe Asthma

Clinical estimates of asthma severity based solely on a patient's interview and examination can result in either an over-estimation or under-estimation of disease severity. For example, loud, audible wheezing is usually a sign of moderate asthma, whereas no wheezing can be an ominous sign associated with severe airflow obstruction.

Symptoms of severe asthma include a sensation of air hunger, severe chest tightness, cough (sometimes productive of sputum but sometimes not), severe fatigue, inability to lie flat in bed, and insomnia. Signs of severe asthma include the use of accessory muscles during respiration, wheezing, an apprehensive appearance, diaphoresis, inability to complete sentences (monosyllabic speech), and difficulty in lying down during the examination. Altered mental status with or without cyanosis is a particularly ominous sign and necessitates immediate emergency care and/or hospitalization. A

Table 4-1   Risk Factors for Near-Fatal and Fatal Asthma

1. Previous history of severe exacerbation requiring admission to an intensive care unit setting, particularly respiratory failure requiring intubation and mechanical ventilation

2. Multiple emergency room visits and/or hospitalizations

3. Overuse of short-acting inhaled bronchodilators

4. Inadequate recognition of the severity of airway obstruction by the patient and/or physician

5. Recent withdrawal of patient from systemic corticosteroids

6. Failure to use anti-inflammatory drugs as primary therapy

7. Poor compliance by the patient

8. Psychiatric or socio-economic problems

9. Extreme variations in peak flow determinations

10. Allergy to *Alternaria* (a mold)

11. Adolescent or elderly patient

12. Limited access to or education about appropriate health care

detailed examination of the chest is necessary, one that looks for signs and symptoms of pneumonia, pneumothorax, or a pneumomediastinum. Many times the last can be suspected by palpating subcutaneous crepitations, especially in the supraclavicular areas of the chest wall.

During the physical examination, special attention should be paid to the patient's blood pressure, pulse, and respiratory rate. Patients with severe asthma usually have a rapid pulse and respiratory rate and an abnormal pulsus paradoxus. A pulsus paradoxus is caused by large swings in intrathoracic pressure and worsens with asthma severity. It is defined as the difference in systolic blood pressure taken between inspiration and expiration. Normally this drop is not greater than 10 mm Hg. A pulsus paradoxus of 10 to 20 mm Hg occurs with moderate airway obstruction, whereas a pulsus paradoxus of >25 mm Hg occurs in severe asthma (3,4).

The symptoms and signs of severe asthma are listed in Table 4-2.

Physiologic and Laboratory Parameters

Serial measurements of lung function allow for the quantification of the severity of airflow obstruction and its response to treatment. Peak expiratory flow (PEF) should be measured in all patients with asthma at each office visit. It offers a quick, simple, and cost-effective means of accurately assessing the severity of airway obstruction.

With the patient standing upright or, if necessary, sitting, he or she is instructed to take a deep breath to maximum inspiration, hold that breath,

Table 4-2   Symptoms and Signs of Severe Asthma

1. Respiratory rate >30 breaths/min

2. Heart rate >120 beats/min

3. Pulsus paradoxus >25 mm Hg

4. Use of accessory muscles of respiration

5. Diaphoresis

6. Inability to complete sentences; monosyllabic speech

7. Inability to lie down during examination

8. Altered mental status

9. Chest examination devoid of wheezing (because of severe airway obstruction)

10. Peak expiratory flow rate <50% of predicted

11. Oxygen saturation <90% with room air

seal lips around a mouthpiece, and blow out as hard and fast as possible. A recording is made and the maneuver repeated twice, with the best of the three recordings logged as the PEF. Coughing into the device can lead to an erroneous high determination. Predicted normal values are based on gender, height, and age (Table 4-3) (5,6). The PEF determination obtained during an asthma exacerbation can be compared with readings obtained at home or with previous readings recorded in the office. The same commercial PEF meter ideally should be used, because there are subtle differences in results when comparing one device with another.

A PEF of <50% predicted or personal best is consistent with a severe exacerbation; 50% to 80% predicted or personal best is consistent with a moderate exacerbation; and >80% predicted or personal best is consistent with a mild exacerbation.

A spirometer is a device for measuring the volume of air exhaled over time. Spirometry measurements can be obtained even in the acutely ill asthmatic by asking the patient to forcibly exhale from the point of maximal inhalation into the spirometer, ideally over 6 seconds. If possible, three determinations should be obtained and the best of the three recorded on the chart.

The forced expiratory volume in 1 second (FEV_1) is the most sensitive test to characterize the degree of airflow obstruction. FEV_1 has much less variability than PEF. In contrast to PEF, FEV_1 is independent of effort once a moderate effort has been made by the patient.

Prediction equations based on studies of large populations of normal subjects have been developed by a number of investigators and are available in standard pulmonary textbooks. Pulmonary function values are expressed as a percent of the predicted value. The physician can therefore compare the patient's pulmonary function with that of the reference population, correlate this with the patient's clinical progress, and make an appropriate assessment.

Table 4-3   Normal Predicted Average Peak Expiratory Flow (PEF) (in L/min)

Age (yrs)	MEN Height (in.)				
	60	65	70	75	80
15	511	531	548	564	578
20	554	575	594	611	626
25	580	603	622	640	656
30	594	617	637	655	672
35	599	622	643	661	677
40	597	620	641	659	675
45	591	613	633	651	668
50	580	602	622	640	656
55	566	588	608	625	640
60	551	572	591	607	622
65	533	554	572	588	603
70	515	535	552	568	582
75	496	515	532	547	560

Age (yrs)	WOMEN Height (in.)				
	55	60	65	70	75
15	423	438	451	463	473
20	444	460	474	486	497
25	455	471	485	497	509
30	458	475	489	502	513
35	458	474	488	501	512
40	453	469	483	496	507
45	446	462	476	488	400
50	437	453	466	478	489
55	427	442	455	467	477
60	415	430	443	454	464
65	403	417	430	441	451
70	390	404	416	427	436
75	377	391	402	413	422

The PEF and FEV_1 percent predicted values are not equivalent or interchangeable and should not be substituted one for the other. Of the two tests, PEF is easier for the patient and more cost effective, FEV_1 the more sensitive (6).

Treatment is not only based on the spirometric determinations but on the clinical findings and previous treatment. For example, a seasonal exacerbation that occurs in a tree-pollen sensitive individual during the spring, when trees pollinate, is usually more easily remedied than is an exacerbation caused by a viral respiratory tract infection. The allergic patient usually responds immediately to inhaled beta-agonist therapy and to an appropriate adjustment in an inhaled corticosteroid, whereas the infected patient is more likely to need a systemic corticosteroid (Case 4-1). Likewise, an individual who is experiencing moderate-to-severe asthma and is overusing a

---

CASE 4-1   *Patient with mild asthma and a respiratory infection who progresses to severe asthma*

A 42-year-old female day care worker has a history of mild intermittent asthma. She developed a persistent cough, facial discomfort, and purulent nasal secretions 10 days after contracting an upper respiratory tract infection. Her asthma had worsened, and she reported only modest improvement with an albuterol metered dose inhaler (MDI).

Her peak expiratory flow (PEF) was 315 L/min, 70% of predicted. Pus was visible in both nares. Lung auscultation revealed a few scattered end-expiratory wheezes.

Initial treatment included amoxicillin and clavulanic acid, 875 mg, twice daily by mouth for 10 days; intranasal aqueous triamcinolone, 55 µg/puff, 2 puffs each nostril daily; and albuterol MDI, 90 µg/puff, 2 puffs, as needed, every 4 hr.

Two days later she returned complaining of increasingly severe shortness of breath, chest tightness, and poor response to the albuterol MDI. Her PEF was 220 L/min, 50% of predicted, and her conversation was repeatedly interrupted by paroxysms of cough. Lung examination revealed diffuse inspiratory and expiratory wheezes. She was given albuterol, 0.5 mg in 3 cc of saline by nebulization, every 20 minutes × 3, and prednisone, 40 mg by mouth. Over the next hour, her PEF improved to 360 L/min, and she had fewer inspiratory and expiratory wheezes. She was discharged on prednisone, 20 mg tid PO for 7 days, and albuterol MDI, 2 puffs every 4 hr, and asked to return in 7 days. She reported by telephone the next day that she was improved. She had diminished frequency and severity of cough and wheeze.

One week later, her PEF was 410, the purulent nasal secretions had dissipated, and lung auscultation revealed only a rare expiratory wheeze with forced expiration. She was placed on inhaled budesonide, 800 µg twice daily, and was asked to maintain this treatment until seen 6 weeks later. Prednisone was discontinued, and she was maintained on the albuterol MDI on an as-needed basis.

Discussion

This case demonstrates that patients with mild asthma can quickly become severely ill when they develop a respiratory tract infection and have concomitant acute sinusitis. An antibiotic was indicated for treatment of acute sinusitis. Prednisone was prescribed when the patient's PEF dropped to <50% of predicted. The earlier use of a high-dose inhaled corticosteroid or oral prednisone may have prevented the more severe asthma. A long-acting beta-agonist may enhance the effectiveness of the inhaled glucocorticoid.

short-acting beta-agonist may be somewhat or completely refractory to nebulized albuterol and generally needs a systemic corticosteroid. Also of importance is the experience the physician has with treating each individual patient. Some patients, particularly severe asthmatics, need a systemic corticosteroid whenever they exacerbate, whereas others can be treated successfully with higher than FDA recommended doses of an inhaled corticosteroid.

Chest radiographs are usually not necessary for the diagnosis of acute asthma, particularly when the physical examination of the chest reveals no unusual findings. However, if the physician suspects a complication, such as pneumonia, pneumothorax, pneumomediastinum, or atelectasis (secondary to mucous plugging), a radiograph should be obtained. When a complication exists, appropriate treatment and close outpatient observation or hospitalization are indicated.

Treatment Strategies

The steps in the management of acute asthma are outlined in Figure 4-1. Recommended doses of asthma medications are summarized in Table 4-4.

Albuterol and Levalbuterol

Treatment should begin with nebulizing albuterol, 2.5 to 5.0 mg, in normal saline, 2.5 to 3.0 cc. This therapy can be repeated as necessary every 20 min until the patient is stable or a decision to hospitalize has been made. The nebulizer may be powered by oxygen, if available, during a severe exacerbation. The first dose of albuterol usually produces the greatest change in pulmonary function; additional doses provide a cumulative effect. However, even high intermittent or continuous doses of albuterol for some patients may have minimal effect because of severe airway obstruction and can result in elevated serum albuterol levels, hypokalemia, and, rarely, cardiac toxicity.

The regular use of any short-acting beta-agonist may result in asthma that is less responsive to its bronchodilatory effects. Albuterol (RS-albuterol) is a racemic mixture of equal parts of the R and S isomers. Some of its adverse effects are thought to be due to the S isomer of the racemic product. The R isomer of albuterol is responsible for the bronchodilatory effects, tachycardia and tremor. It is rapidly metabolized and achieves lower peak concentrations and has a shorter half-life than the S isomer. The S isomer does not bind to the beta-receptor nor does it cause bronchodilation. *In vitro* it increases intracellular calcium in smooth muscle cells and causes muscle cell shortening, thereby theoretically enhancing contractile responses. The S isomer may also induce airway hyperresponsiveness to a variety of nonspecific agents or allergens and may have proinflammatory effects. As a result of these *in vitro* studies, it has been suggested that

Assess Asthma Severity

- Measure PEF: If <50% personal best or predicted, severe asthma is suggested
- Note signs and symptoms of asthma: degree of cough, breathlessness, wheeze (may not correlate well with severity of asthma), use of accessory muscles, and suprasternal retractions

Initial Treatment: Albuterol, 90 µg/puff, 2 to 4 puffs, by metered dose inhaler with or without a spacer, as necessary, *or* albuterol, 2.5 to 5.0 mg in 2.5 to 3 cc, saline, single, nebulization treatment every 20 min for up to 3 doses or continuously if necessary

Assess Response

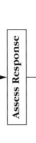

Good Response (Mild Episode)

- PEF >80% personal best or predicted
- No wheezing or shortness of breath; patient becomes asymptomatic
- Response to beta-2 agonist treatment sustained for 4 hr

Incomplete Response (Moderate Episode)

- PEF = 50% to 80% personal best or predicted
- Persistent wheezing or shortness of breath

Prednisone, 20 mg q 8–12 hr, *or* high-dose inhaled corticosteroid such as fluticasone, 220 µg/puff, 2 or 3 puffs 4 times daily, or budesonide, 200 µg/puff, 4 or 5 puffs 4 times daily; any inhaled corticosteroid can be used by doubling or tripling the usual recommended dose

Poor Response (Severe Episode)

- PEF <50% personal best or predicted and does not improve
- Marked inspiratory and expiratory wheezing and shortness of breath; absence of wheeze may suggest that patient has extreme asthma and that respiratory arrest may occur

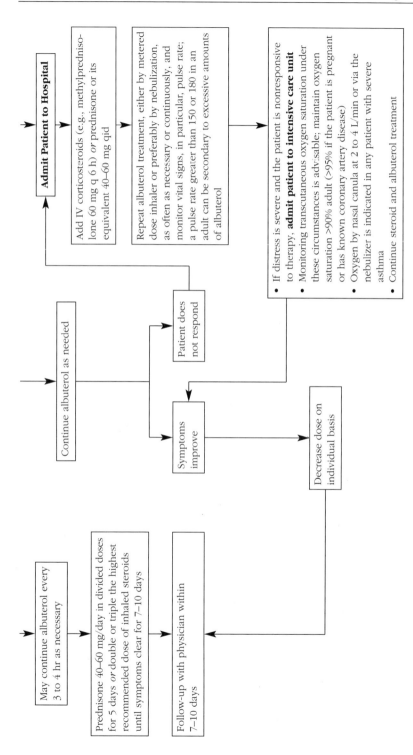

Figure 4-1   Algorithm for the management of acute asthma.

Table 4-4   Dosages of Drugs for Asthma Exacerbations

Inhaled short-acting beta-2 agonists

Albuterol

Nebulizer solution (5 mg/mL)	2.5–5.0 mg every 20 min for 1 hr, then 2.5–10 mg every 1 to 4 hr as needed, or 10–15 mg/hr continuously; "drive" nebulizer with oxygen
MDI (90 mcg/puff)	4–8 puffs every 20 min for up to 4 hr, then every 1–4 hr as needed, with or without spacer
Levalbuterol HCl nebulizer solution (0.63 mg)	0.63 mgs every 6–8 hr, may be increased to 1.25 mgs every 6–8 hr for those with more severe symptoms not responding to 0.63 mg

Systemic (injected) beta-2 agonists

Epinephrine 1:1000 w/v (1 mg/mL)	0.2–0.3 mg subcutaneously every 20 min for 3 doses (for patients with severe asthma; unable or unwilling to use MDI/spacer or nebulizer); higher doses of epinephrine can be used as necessary

Anticholinergics

Ipratropium bromide nebulizer solution (0.25 mg/mL)	0.5 mg every 30 min for 3 doses, then every 2–4 hr as needed; may mix with albuterol solution; not considered a first-line therapy; should be added to albuterol therapy
MDI (18 µg/puff)	4 puffs every 30 min for 3 doses, then every 2–4 hr as needed

Corticosteroids

Prednisone, prednisolone	For outpatient "burst" use 45–60 mg in 3 divided doses for as long as necessary
Methylprednisolone	36–48 mg in 3 divided doses for as long as necessary
Metered dose inhaled	Double or triple the highest recommended dose for 7–10 days or as long as necessary
Budesonide solution	0.25 or 0.5 mg/mL nebules; mixing with other medications not recommended

Adapted from the National Heart, Lung and Blood Institute. Guidelines for the Diagnosis and Management of Asthma. Expert Panel Report No. 2. US Department of Health and Human Services; July 1997.

continued administration of racemic albuterol and accumulation of the S isomer may contribute to worsening of asthma and account for the lack of clinical efficacy of this medication in some patients.

An alternative to albuterol, particularly in the severe asthmatic who is overusing a short-acting beta-agonist, is levalbuterol, the active R isomer of racemic albuterol. It also is used to treat acute asthma. It has been suggested that by removing the S isomer, levalbuterol, a third-generation beta-agonist, retains the clinical benefit of racemic albuterol without potential detrimental side effects. Levalbuterol can be used for all patients as first-line therapy for acute asthma. Approved for ages 12 and above, the duration of action of levalbuterol HCl solution in studies is approximately 5 to 8 hr. However, in the author's experience, it can be used repeatedly (as can albuterol) for treatment of acute asthma. Drug compatibility, efficacy, and safety of levalbuterol, when mixed with other drugs via nebulization, have not been established; however, there is no reason to believe that levalbuterol should not be mixed with other solutions. The usual starting dose, 0.63 mg in 3 cc unit dosages, has reduced systemic beta-agonist side effects compared with albuterol 2.5 mg. The highest levalbuterol dose recommended is 1.25 mg in a 3 cc solution. Levalbuterol is approved for use every 6 to 8 hr. Though more expensive than albuterol, levalbuterol may have an improved therapeutic index, but more studies are necessary to determine whether levalbuterol is more effective than albuterol for the treatment of acute asthma (7).

Ipratropium Bromide

Ipratropium bromide is a quaternary derivative of atropine available as a solution for nebulization and provides competitive inhibition of acetylcholine at the muscarinic cholinergic receptor, thereby relaxing smooth muscle in large, central airways. It is used to treat severe asthma, especially when albuterol is not optimally beneficial. Ipratropium bromide, 0.5 mg in 2.5 cc, is added to the unit dose of albuterol and administered every 20 min for three doses, then every 2 to 4 hr as needed. It is not recommended for use alone (i.e., without albuterol) for treatment of acute asthma. There are no data for its use with levalbuterol; however, there is no reason to expect that its efficacy would be different than when combined with albuterol (8).

Epinephrine

If the patient is not responding to albuterol, levalbuterol, and/or ipratropium bromide, epinephrine, 1:1000 w/v, 0.2 to 0.3 cc, given subcutaneously in the arm every 20 min for several doses, can be tried as long as the patient is carefully monitored for signs of adrenergic toxicity. If there is no immediate response to epinephrine, it should be discontinued and the patient hospitalized.

Methylxanthines

Aminophylline and theophylline are methylxanthines that have been used for the treatment of asthma for over 65 years. Before the advent of more selective beta-adrenergic drugs and inhaled anti-inflammatory agents methylxanthines were used as first-line therapy for treatment of acute as well as chronic stable asthma. Because of their narrow therapeutic window, increased incidence of side effects, numerous drug-drug interactions, and the need to monitor serum levels, methylxanthines are no longer used as first-line therapy to treat acute or chronic asthma.

There are conflicting reports regarding whether methylxanthines are efficacious for treatment of acute asthma. Some clinical trials indicate that intravenous aminophylline may be useful, especially when the patient is refractory to more conventional therapy. Because aminophylline is rarely used at this time for treatment of acute asthma, the treating physician must be aware of drug interactions, clinical situations that warrant adjustments in the dose, and monitoring of therapy. For most adult nonsmokers the aminophylline dose is 5 to 6 mg/kg slowly IV over 20 to 30 min followed by a maintenance dose of 0.4 mg/kg/hr. The dose should be adjusted to 0.6 mg/kg/hr for smokers and to 0.2 mg/kg/hr for patients with congestive heart failure or liver disease. The serum concentration, to be determined every 4 to 6 hr after initiating treatment, should be maintained at 10 to 15 µg/mL. Serum concentrations of theophylline above 20 µg/mL are considered to be toxic and are associated with a high incidence of nausea, vomiting, headache, and even cardiac effects (9).

Corticosteroids

Many patients with asthma with mild, moderate, or sometimes even severe exacerbations of asthma can be successfully treated using a higher than recommended dose of an inhaled corticosteroid regardless of whether they are already taking an inhaled corticosteroid (Case 4-2). For example, the dose of fluticasone may be increased from a top maintenance dose of 440 µg bid to 440 µg 4x/day or even 660 µg 4x/day for a flare-up of asthma. The dose of budesonide may be increased from 800 µg 2x/day as a top maintenance up to 800 µg 4x/day or even up to 1000 µg 4x/day. Other investigators suggest that inhaled budesonide, 1600 µg twice daily, via dry powder inhaler, may be an alternative to oral systemic prednisolone for acute asthma (10). Any inhaled corticosteroid can be used in this fashion by doubling or tripling the highest recommended dose.

The most opportune moment to use high-dose inhaled corticosteroids is before the patient becomes too ill to continue management at home. Asthma exacerbations may respond to such therapy, therefore obviating the need for systemic corticosteroids. Use of a high-dose inhaled corticosteroid decreases potential side effects (e.g., insomnia, increased appetite, hyperactivity) associated with an oral corticosteroid, not to mention the potential detrimental effects on bone metabolism and other organ systems (11).

Higher doses of inhaled corticosteroids are less likely to work in patients who are overusing their beta-agonist and in those patients who have

CASE 4-2   *Patient with acute asthma caused by exposure to allergen*

A 52-year-old male with a life-long history of asthma and allergic rhinitis has required inhaled fluticasone 110, 2 puffs bid, and salmeterol (a long-acting beta-agonist), 2 puffs bid, to control his asthma. He is self-employed and works from his home. Prick puncture skin tests with aeroallergens were highly positive to dust mites and cat. Avoidance measures, loratadine 10 mg daily, and a continuation of his previous asthma medication resulted in adequate control of symptoms.

This spring he was asked by his daughter, a college student, to care for her cat and two new kittens while away on spring break. Eager to comply, he prepared an area in the den for his new guests. Within the first several hours of their arrival, he reported increasing frequency of sneeze, cough, and wheeze, especially while working in his den. His symptoms were becoming increasingly difficult to control with a short-acting beta-adrenergic inhaler used on a prn basis.

Review of peak flow rates recorded while at home revealed a consistent drop to around 450 L/min, 75% of his personal best, during morning and afternoon hours. Peak expiratory flow rates improved to normal on weekends when he was at his oceanside condominium without the cats. His examination was unremarkable except for a clear, watery discharge from both nostrils, nasal pallor and edema, and minimal wheezing.

He was advised to increase the fluticasone to 220 μg, 3 puffs tid, and continue salmeterol, 2 puffs bid, loratadine, and add albuterol MDI, 2 puffs every 4 hr as needed. His physician suggested that the cats be removed from the home as soon as possible.

Within 2 weeks of the cats' departure, he reported marked improvement. A review of his recorded PEFs revealed a consistent upward trend to a personal best of 600 L/min. The higher dose inhaled fluticasone, 220 μg, 3 puffs bid, was reduced to 2 puffs bid for several weeks and thereafter to 1 puff bid, and all other medications were continued. He now rarely needs to use albuterol MDI.

Discussion

This case illustrates the importance of allergens in exacerbating this patient's chronic asthma and allergic rhinitis. Recognizing a drop in PEF at home can be important; the physician is able to objectively determine that the worsening asthma is most likely secondary to exposure to an indoor etiology, in this case cat allergen.

---

severe upper respiratory tract infections exacerbating their asthma. A systemic corticosteroid usually is necessary in these patients. Long-term use of a systemic corticosteroid may result in suppression of the hypothalamic-pituitary-adrenal (HPA) axis. For patients who are receiving long-term or frequent bursts of systemic corticosteroid therapy, close observation for signs of adrenal insufficiency is advised, especially as the systemic corticosteroid is gradually tapered and the patient is transferred to an inhaled corticosteroid. Under these circumstances, a brief period using both a systemic and an inhaled corticosteroid is advised to assure asthma control, lessen withdrawal side effects, and permit the HPA axis to begin to function normally, although it may take a full year off systemic corticosteroids before that occurs. If a patient has received high-dose systemic corticosteroid therapy for more than several weeks during the previous year, he or she is considered at-risk for adrenal insufficiency associated with stress (e.g., a serious illness, pneumonia, general surgery) and should be given a systemic corticosteroid at this time.

A study in hospitalized adults with asthma (PEF of 33% to 70% predicted) compared high-dose nebulized budesonide suspension, 4 mg q 8h for 48 hr, followed by a tapering dose of budesonide Turbuhaler (initially 1600 µg bid for 7 days, then 800 µg bid an additional 21 days) for 28 days total, with oral prednisolone, 40 mg by mouth for 9 to 11 days, followed by a moderate dose of budesonide Turbuhaler, 800 µg bid for 21 days, and found that both regimens were successful in treating acute asthma. Nebulized corticosteroids may assist in regaining control of symptoms during an exacerbation of asthma (12).

Following office treatment, the patient must be instructed to repeatedly measure his or her peak flow and be aware of worsening symptoms. The patient must also be followed closely by the physician with appropriate follow-up office visits, usually every 7 to 10 days initially, then, when stable, every several months.

Short courses or "bursts" of systemic corticosteroids are effective for establishing control when initiating therapy for severe asthma or during a period of gradual deterioration not responding to higher doses of an inhaled corticosteroid. Prednisone or its equivalent, 45 to 60 mg/day, in three divided doses is recommended. The burst should be continued until the patient is well or achieves a PEF of 80% of their personal or predicted best. Most patients respond rapidly and are considerably improved in 5 days, whereas others may take up to 10 to 14 days to respond. Corticosteroid-resistant patients with asthma may take weeks to respond, and some eventually need a systemic corticosteroid on a daily or every-other-day basis to supplement their inhaled corticosteroid.

Tapering the dose of systemic corticosteroids after a short course (less than 1 week) is unnecessary. Oral corticosteroids can be stopped and an inhaled corticosteroid started at high doses. When systemic corticosteroids are used longer than 10 to 14 days, it is advisable to taper the medication over days or a week or two because tapering seems to lessen the post-corticosteroid side effects (e.g., depression, fatigue, myalgias, arthralgias). Some doctors use an IM corticosteroid as initial treatment for acute asthma; however, there is no scientific evidence that injectable IM or even IV corticosteroids have a more rapid onset of action than does an oral corticosteroid. IM or IV corticosteroids may be more advisable when the patient is severely dyspneic, noncompliant, or has nausea or vomiting associated with an asthma exacerbation.

Leukotriene Modifying Agents

Leukotrienes are proinflammatory mediators involved in the pathogenesis of asthma. Leukotriene modifying agents have a rapid onset of action and improve the FEV_1 within 1 to 2 hr following ingestion in patients with chronic asthma. They are currently under study for treatment of acute asthma.

Antibiotics

Antibiotics are usually not indicated for acute asthma because most exacerbations are secondary to viral respiratory tract infections, chronic or acute exposures to allergens, or exposure to irritants. However, antibiotics are indicated with acute suppurative sinusitis, with a concomitant bacterial pneumonia, or when bacterial infection is suspect. Influenza vaccine yearly and Pneumovax every 5 to 6 years are indicated in all patients with asthma.

Hospitalization

Failure to respond to office treatment or subsequent deterioration dictates hospitalization, usually in an intensive care unit. The patient should be hydrated with IV fluids or, if possible, orally, and administered oxygen, 2 to 4 L/min via a nasal cannula, then followed with telemetry and pulse oximetery. Repeat blood gas determinations are made until the patient is stable. The patient should be treated with continuous nebulization of albuterol or levalbuterol with or without ipratropium bromide and high-dose corticosteroids such as methylprednisolone, 1 to 2 mg/kg, or its equivalent for 24 hr, in divided doses every 8 hr, either intravenously or orally. Consultation with an asthma specialist is indicated at this time. If the patient is not responding to inpatient treatment and is deteriorating, a decision should be made to assist ventilation before the patient has a respiratory arrest.

Avoiding Severe Asthma

Patients with asthma rarely need emergency care or hospitalization. Serious asthma exacerbations usually can be avoided by appropriate prevention, education, and treatment (Case 4-3). The patient should have adequate knowledge of the pathophysiology of asthma (i.e., asthma is a chronic disease that necessitates the avoidance of allergens and prevention of infections, the appropriate use of medications, PEF determinations, and early

CASE 4-3   *Patient with chronic intermittently severe asthma, nasal polyps, and aspirin intolerance*

A 37-year-old male with a history of chronic intermittently severe asthma, aspirin and other nonsteroidal anti-inflammatory drug intolerance, and nasal polyps develops a sudden onset of severe cough and chest tightness after walking 2 miles to his home on a dry cold day. His past medical history is remarkable for poor medication compliance, three hospitalizations with two ICU admissions, and at least four urgent care evaluations for acute asthma within the past 20 months. On these last occasions, he is treated in an emergency room and discharged on a short course of an oral corticosteroid for 7 to 10 days. He is unable to identify a primary care physician.

The patient's current medications include an over-the-counter bronchodilator and an "herbal remedy" for asthma. He is reluctant to take any more "steroids" because of a fear of side effects of insomnia and weight gain.

In the office he is barely able to perform a PEF test. He is using accessory muscles to breath and talks in monosyllabic sentences. He has generalized decreased breath sounds, and a few expiratory wheezes are heard.

An IV is started, and he is rapidly hydrated with 5% glucose in water. He is given oxygen, 4 L/min, by nasal cannula and nebulized albuterol, 0.5 mg in 3 cc of saline over 20 min. He becomes more apprehensive and complains of "claustrophobia". Epinephrine, 1:1000 w/v, 0.3 cc, is given SQ and results in some improvement. Intravenous methylprednisolone, 40 mg, is administered over 5 min. A second dose of epinephrine, 0.3 cc, is administered 15 min later while nebulized albuterol is continued. He is transferred by ambulance to the ICU, and an asthma specialist is consulted. Appropriate blood gas determinations and laboratory studies are ordered. The patient is continued on oxygen; IV methylprednisolone, 40 mg q 8 hr; nebulized albuterol; and IV fluids. Five days later, he is discharged on a tapering dose of prednisone; budesonide, 800 µg, twice daily; salmeterol, 2 puffs, twice daily; and MDI albuterol on a prn basis.

The patient subsequently sees a specialist, is scheduled for skin tests, and is being considered for aspirin desensitization, known to benefit from one-third to one-half of patients with the aspirin triad (aspirin and other nonsteroidal anti-inflammatory drug intolerance, asthma, and nasal polyposis and/or chronic sinusitis). He will also be placed on a leukotriene receptor antagonist during aspirin desensitization and thereafter continued on this medication. Intranasal fluticasone, 50 µg/spray, 2 sprays in each nostril daily, will be used to control his nasal polyps.

Discussion

This case illustrates the importance of recognizing a patient at risk for fatal asthma. Frequent use of an emergency room, recent hospitalizations, lack of compliance, and the use of over-the-counter remedies in a patient with complex disease, all contributed to his life-threatening events. Education and follow-up care with a specialist are of utmost importance in preventing future exacerbations.

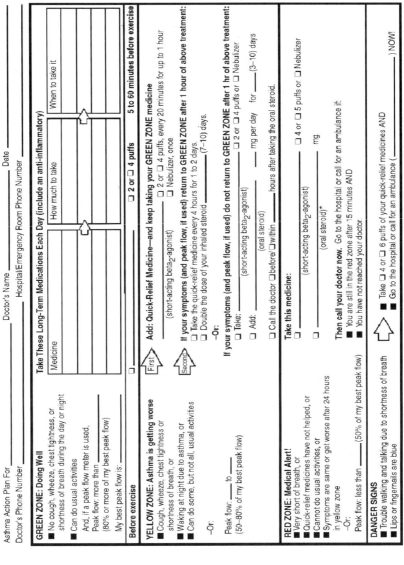

Figure 4-2 Example of an "Asthma Action Plan." These written instructions help the patient initiate and carry out proper asthma management in the event of an exacerbation until the physician can be reached. These instructions can also be used to remind the patient about the day-to-day management of chronic asthma. (From National Heart, Lung and Blood Institute. National Asthma Education and Prevention Program; NIH Publication No. 97-4053; the footnote has been added editorially [2002].)

recognition of an impending exacerbation). When an exacerbation is likely, the patient should have a "back-up" program available to initiate on his or her own and at the same time contact the physician (Fig. 4-2). Early use of either increased doses of an inhaled corticosteroid or initiation of oral corticosteroids is imperative in such cases. The patient should also be instructed to increase the use of short-acting beta-agonists, as often as every half-hour or hour, until the physician can be contacted for additional help, or, if necessary, go to an emergency room.

The physician should be made aware by telephone about the exacerbation and examine the patient as soon as possible. Open communication between the physician and patient, a written action plan, ongoing assessment, and modification of the treatment regimen, as necessary, form the essential foundation for a successful partnership for asthma care (13).

⬛   ⬛   ⬛

Key Points

- Physicians should be aware of the risk factors for fatal and near-fatal asthma and the importance of early recognition and treatment of acute asthma.

- In addition to the history and physical examination, pulmonary function testing is used to assess asthma severity. A PEF of less than 50% predicted or personal best indicates severe asthma, a PEF of 50% to 80% predicted indicates moderate asthma, and a PEF of more than 80% predicted indicates mild asthma.

- Initial treatment of acute asthma is albuterol 2.5 to 5.0 mg in 2.5 to 3 mL saline every 20 min until the patient is stable.

- Mild, moderate, and sometimes even severe exacerbations of asthma can be successfully treated by using a higher than recommended dose of an inhaled corticosteroid, sometimes increased by as much as two or three times the recommended dose.

⬛   ⬛   ⬛

REFERENCES

1. **National Heart, Lung and Blood Institute.** Guidelines for the diagnosis and management of asthma. Expert Panel Report No. 2. US Department of Health and Human Services; July 1997.

2. **Guishard K.** Fatal asthma. In: Brenner BE, ed. Emergency Asthma. New York: Marcel Dekker; 1999:273–87.

3. **Town GI.** Diagnosis in adults. In: Busse WW, Holgate ST, eds. Asthma and Rhinitis, 2nd ed. London: Blackwell Science; 2000:1735–73.

4. **Corbridge T, Hall JB.** Critical care management. In: Busse WW, Holgate ST, eds. Asthma and Rhinitis, 2nd ed. London: Blackwell Science; 2000:1848–63.

5. **Nunn AJ, Gregg I.** New regression equations for predicting peak expiratory flow in adults. BMJ. 1989;298:1068–70.

6. **Silverman R, Scharf SM.** Pulmonary function testing in the emergency department. In: Brenner BE, ed. Emergency Asthma. New York: Marcel Dekker; 1999:233–52.

7. **Nelson HS, Bensch G, Pleskow WW, et al.** Improved bronchodilation with levalbuterol compared with racemic albuterol in patients with asthma. J Allergy Clin Immunol. 1998;102:943–52.

8. **Rodrigo G, Rodrigo C, Burschtin O.** A meta-analysis of the effects of ipratropium bromide in adults with acute asthma. Am J Med. 1999;107:363–70.

9. **Madison JM, Irwin R.** Status asthmaticus. In: Irwin RS, Cerra FB, Rippe JM, eds. Intensive Care Management, 4th ed. Philadelphia: Lippincott-Raven; 1999:592–606.

10. **Nana A, Youngchaiyud P, Charoenratanakul S, et al.** High dose inhaled budesonide may substitute for oral therapy after an acute attack of asthma. J Asthma. 1998;35:647–55.

11. **Tan RA, Spector SL.** High dose inhaled steroids. In: Williams PV, ed. Immunology and Allergy Clinics of North America. Philadelphia: WB Saunders; 1996;16:765–76.

12. **Higenbottom TW, Britton J, Lawrence D, et al.** Comparison of nebulized budesonide and prednisolone in severe asthma exacerbation in adults. BioDrugs. 2000;14:247–54.

13. **Lockey RF.** The basic principles of asthma management today. J Respir Dis. 1998;19(suppl):S7–13.

5

Environmental Controls in the Management of Asthma

Saba Samee, MD

Thomas A. E. Platts-Mills, MD

Large numbers of patients present to their primary care physicians with symptoms of asthma, allergic rhinitis, or atopic dermatitis. The management of these conditions is multifold but should include consideration of reducing exposure to the allergens that can play a central role in these chronic inflammatory diseases. Seasonal symptoms are usually caused by the pollen of trees (February-April), grasses (May-June), or ragweed (August-September). In addition, outdoor mold spore exposure plays an important role in both allergic rhinitis and asthma; however, it is now well recognized that exposure to allergens indoors plays the dominant role in perennial allergic disease.

Although many different indoor allergens can contribute to allergic rhinitis and asthma (e.g., rodents, spiders, ladybugs, various species of molds, many different pets), the best-defined sources are dust mites, cats, dogs, and the German cockroach. Environmental control presents a challenge, because it can be difficult to find practical and effective methods of reducing exposure to allergens. Allergen-specific avoidance has been shown to be beneficial for symptomatic patients with evidence of specific immediate sensitivity. Although the patient's symptoms may provide clues, a clear correlation between exposure to allergens and perennial asthma symptoms is generally not evident. Therefore, patients with chronic symptoms should either be skin tested or have blood tests to evaluate for specific IgE antibodies to aeroallergens. When the cause is identified, allergen avoidance should be included as part of first-line therapy.

The significance of house dust in asthma was first recognized by Kern in 1921 when he and others talked about advising patients to control dust exposure. Interestingly, when Rackeman defined *intrinsic* asthma in 1947, a key feature was that patients "didn't get better in hospital." He recognized that the improvement in asthma symptoms in hospital was in large part due to decreasing extrinsic allergen exposure. When we demonstrated that decreased bronchial hyperreactivity (BHR) to histamine could also be achieved by moving mite-allergic patients into allergen-free hospital rooms in London (1), it was clear that decreased BHR should be the objective of avoidance treatment. In that study, the air in the rooms was passed through high-efficiency particulate air (HEPA) filters, the rooms had polished floors, and mite allergen decreased from 13.7 µg/g at home to <0.2 µg/g in the hospital rooms. This study confirmed the effectiveness of allergen avoidance outside of the home but the question became: Could these conditions be achieved at home?

An attempt to measure the clinical efficacy of biologically significant mite allergen avoidance at home in children with asthma and dust-mite hypersensitivity was performed by Ehnert et al (2). They demonstrated the superiority of an encasing regimen whereby mattresses, pillows, and comforters were covered in cotton encasings coated on one side with polyurethane versus the use of chemicals including an acaricide (benzyl benzoate) on mattresses and carpets. The encasing group experienced a significant decrease in BHR, as judged by the reactivity of the lungs to histamine (PC_{20} increased 4.5-fold over 8 months), as well as a 91% decrease in mite-allergen exposure (<2 µg/g of mattress dust within 14 days). This demonstrated that environmental control measures such as encasings could be safe, effective, nontoxic, and practicable. Avoidance has been shown to decrease BHR and to decrease asthma symptoms and medication use. Recent studies confirm that dust mite allergen can be significantly reduced in homes utilizing various methods, resulting in asthma improvement as demonstrated by a decrease in BHR (3). The goal of this chapter is to provide guidelines for the management of environmental allergens in allergic patients.

Dust Mites

Environment

Voorhorst et al are credited with the discovery in 1967 that dust mites (Fig. 5-1, *A*) are the major source of allergen in house dust. In the United States, the most common species are *Dermatophagoides pteronyssinus, D. farinae,* and, to a lesser extent, *Euroglyphus maynei.* Usually one species dominates the total mite population in a home; therefore, allergy testing should test for more than one species (usually *D. pteronyssinus* and *D. farinae*). House dust mites rely on the presence of water in the environment, and they feed on skin scales and other organic debris. With some adjustment for varying temperature, the optimum relative humidity (RH) for mite growth is between 60% and 75%. In humid environments mites can grow anywhere including clothing, drapes, bedding, upholstered furniture, stuffed animals, and carpets. Mite allergen remains airborne for short periods of time and falls quickly. Because air filtration requires particles to remain airborne, its role in mite allergen reduction is unclear.

Methods of Avoidance

Physical Barriers

Initially, weekly vacuuming of mattresses was recommended to control dust mites, but compliance was rare because of its difficulty. When mattress covering was advised, many patients resisted because they believed that placing a mattress in an encasing would lead to the growth of mold and decomposition of the mattress. Furthermore, the initial plastic encasings with zippers were not well tolerated, even though they were very effective in preventing mite allergen exposure. Subsequently, more comfortable fabrics that allowed for air movement but prohibited the leakage of dust were used for encasings. More recently, fine-woven fabrics have been introduced that have a variety of pore sizes enabling varying degrees of airflow. The size can vary from ~2 to 20 μm, with the ease of airflow directly related to pore size. A pore size of 6 to 10 μm allows for little or no mite allergen leakage (Fig. 5-1, B), whereas a pore size of 6 pm prevents leakage of cat allergen (4). With the advent of these fabrics, it is now possible to recommend mattress, box spring, duvet, and pillowcase covers to all allergic patients (Case 5-1). The cost of these covers varies greatly, and patients should be advised of the possible expense. If cost is an issue, one can spend more money on the pillow covers (and perhaps covers on comforters), because these are directly in contact with the skin, whereas less-expensive covers, including plastic covers, can be used for mattresses and box springs.

Washing and Drying of Linens

Further research revealed that dust mites and other allergens were difficult to remove from homes by regular cleaning methods. Simply washing linens, especially with the newer cool-wash detergents, was not sufficiently effective in removing mites or mite allergen. Many studies revealed that the minimum temperature required to kill mites had to be ≥130°F. In fact, hot-water temperature in most homes in the United States is 120°F because of an American Academy of Pediatrics recommendation aimed at reducing the risk of accidental burns in infants and young children. With this in mind, the water temperature in homes should not exceed 130°F. If necessary, linens can be washed in a commercial washer, where the temperature is usually 140°F. Other effective means of killing mites include drying linens outside in the sun or in a tumble dryer at 130°F for at least 20 min. Studies looking at dry cleaning have demonstrated that some methods are effective at killing mites, and some are not.

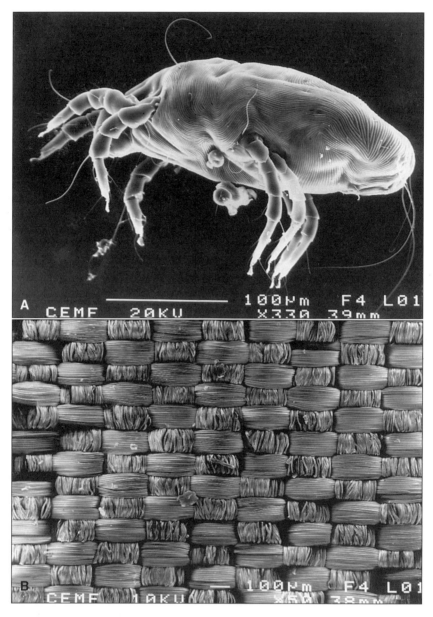

Figure 5-1   Scanning electron micrographs of (A) dust mite and (B) fine-woven fabric (6 μm); the pore size of the fabric does not allow for passage of dust mites. (Courtesy of Bonnie Sheppard and John Vaughan.)

Carpets, Dehumidifiers, and Chemical Agents

Another major reservoir for allergens is carpeting. Until the advent of the vacuum cleaner, it was common practice to only lay carpet down in the

CASE 5-1   *Cleaning and barrier methods that minimize exposure to dust mite allergens*

A 17-year-old female presents for evaluation of nasal congestion, nocturnal coughing, and wheezing. The symptoms get better during the day and recur every evening. She has a history of wheezing with colds but is fairly active. She has a prescription for albuterol prn, which she has not used. Her symptoms are worse in the fall. Her bedroom is on the ground floor and has wall-to-wall carpeting, heavy drapes, and many stuffed animals that sit on her bed.

Physical examination shows an inflamed and boggy nasal mucosa but is otherwise unremarkable. Skin testing is positive for dust mites and cats. Spirometry reveals an FEV_1 of 75%.

After discussion with her parents, they agree to place encasements on her mattress, box springs, and pillows along with regular washing of bed linens in hot water. The patient removes the dust-accumulating items in her bedroom. The physician prescribes a nasal steroid, one spray in each nostril at bedtime for 1 month. She begins an inhaled steroid twice a day and uses the albuterol every 4 hr as needed for wheezing. When she returns one month later, her parents report that she is sleeping well through the night and that she no longer complains of nasal congestion. Her FEV_1 is now 93%.

Discussion

Often, modifications in living conditions are necessary for dust mite allergic patients. Simple changes work to make pharmacologic therapy more effective. Although seasonal variation in dust mite growth does not occur in all parts of the country, it can be very marked, usually peaking from July through November. This variation can often allow a patient to use medications during the months of greatest exposure, thereby minimizing the use of medications when allergen exposure is not clinically significant.

winters and to clean and air the carpets outside on a regular basis. Wall-to-wall carpeting accumulates large amounts of human debris, which provides ample food for mites and other insects. It is difficult to clean carpets thoroughly, even with a vacuum cleaner, because dirt and mites settle deep into the carpet and padding. Nonetheless, a vacuum cleaner remains mandatory for cleaning carpets (see next section).

Along with ample human skin scales for food and optimal indoor temperature for growth (i.e., 65°F to 75°F), ambient humidity plays a key role in dust mite proliferation. Mites best absorb water from the air when the RH is between 60% and 75%. This differentiates dust mites from insects such as cockroaches, which can move around and find water, allowing them to survive in low humidity. This difference is obvious from the low prevalence of dust mites in dry climates (e.g., Arizona, in apartments in the upper Midwest such as Chicago). It has long been recognized that controlling humidity is a potential method of decreasing mite proliferation. Recent studies have shown that using a whole-house dehumidifier that maintains an RH of <51% can be very helpful (5).

Using dehumidifiers and air conditioning can often help reduce humidity. However, newer air conditioning units only cool air to just below the set temperature, thereby removing only minimum amounts of water. Older units would cool to lower temperatures, thereby removing larger amounts of water, which resulted in a lower RH once the air was rewarmed (6).

A variety of chemicals have been recommended for mite eradication in homes. Mites are not insects, and many insecticides do not kill them in the doses that are used in residential areas. The poor penetration of insecticides into thick mattresses, carpets and upholstery adds to this difficulty.

Two chemicals have been studied extensively in mite control: benzyl benzoate and tannic acid. Benzyl benzoate (BB) was developed as a powder by Bischoff in Germany as a combined carpet cleaning agent and acaricide. BB can kill mites (it is also used as a scabicide), has been used as a human food preservative, and is without any reports of toxicity despite widespread use in homes. Thus BB appears ideal for home use. However, the difficulty lies in ensuring that a sufficient quantity of the powder penetrates the thick materials that normally harbor dust mites. There is still debate as to whether BB should be incorporated as a standard method for controlling dust mites. Public perception of strong chemicals sprayed in the home is poor, even more so when there are children and frail individuals at risk for exposure. BB is not currently available in the United States. Recently, compounds containing boron have been marketed for killing dust mites. Preliminary data suggest that they are effective.

Tannic acid (TA) has been used for many centuries as a denaturing agent or protein-stabilizing agent. It is consumed in large quantities (e.g., in tea) and has low oral toxicity. One of its limiting qualities is that TA non-specifically binds proteins such that large quantities of TA are required to denature allergens when other proteins are present. This suggests that the quantity of TA required to remove cat allergens in carpets, with multiple other proteins present, would be too large for consumer use.

Vacuum Cleaners

Wall-to-wall carpeting provides a large reservoir for the accumulation of dust, debris, and dirt. Despite marketing claims, it is extremely difficult for even the most powerful vacuum cleaners to remove live mites and all debris from carpets. Furthermore, faulty connections can allow air laden with allergens to escape. A primary concern in vacuum cleaner design is the amount of allergen that becomes airborne while vacuuming. Studies have shown that most airborne allergen is generated from the exiting airflow rather than from the beating action of the brushes. Double-thickness bags or specially designed nonwoven synthetic materials may improve filtration, but the thickness of the bag does not always predict the effectiveness of the bag. Studies have also shown that the addition of a final filter, including HEPA filters, can eliminate allergen leakage. One can argue that when maximal cleaning of carpets does not alleviate the allergen burden from homes of allergic patients, a polished wood floor should be considered. In cases where there is a concrete slab or an unventilated space, the use of tile, vinyl, or polished wood flooring is preferable. Homes of atopic patients should be designed so that carpets can be removed if there is a symptomatic person at home. In addition, items that accumulate dust should be removed and the symptomatic person should not be in the room for at least 20 min following vacuuming.

Air Cleaners

The lucrative industry of air purification systems is rapidly expanding. Because the air we breathe contains allergens and impurities, the idea of being able to clean it is attractive. It is important to note that both allergic and nonallergic individuals may benefit from removal of irritant particles (e.g., tobacco smoke) from the air.

The goal of air filtration is to efficiently remove particles that are carrying allergens or irritants. The ability of a filter to do this depends on resistance to airflow, efficiency of filtration, and proper maintenance. Simple filtration can be achieved by forcing air through packed fibers; the closer they are, the finer is the filtration. Finely pleated paper or spot-welded nonwoven fibers can be used to trap smaller particles.

The most efficient filters are HEPA filters, which by definition must remove 99.97% of all airborne particles 0.3 µm in size. These filters are often made of minipleated microfine glass paper. Due to their high resistance, HEPA filters should be reserved for room filtration and vacuum cleaners. Another type of filter is the electrostatic filter, which places a charge on airborne particles causing them to adhere to a specific receptacle. Electrostatic filters can be up to 90% effective and have the added benefit of very low resistance. Their use in treating allergic patients has been limited because it is difficult to determine their efficiency of filtration and particle size limitation. They also produce ozone to some degree. Although often mentioned as a means of allergen avoidance, central air duct cleaning in homes has not demonstrated improvement in clinical outcomes.

The present recommendation is to use a HEPA filter for room air filtration, nonwoven filters for heating and air conditioners, and a good-quality two-layered "paper" bag for vacuum cleaners (Table 5-1) (6). Air cleaners are definitely relevant to the management of domestic animal allergy but may also play a secondary role in mite allergy.

Domestic Animals

Approximately 60% of homes in the United States have a domestic animal. These pets produce large amounts of proteins that can be allergenic and

Table 5-1   Indoor Allergens: Characteristics and Avoidance

Allergen	Source/Reservoirs	Airborne	Primary Avoidance Measures
Dust mites (Der p 1 and Der f 1)	• Breed in dark, humid "nests" (e.g., carpets, sofas, mattresses, pillows) • Temperature 60–75°F	• Particles ≥10 µm fall rapidly	• Encasements • Wash in hot water (≥130°F) • Minimize reservoirs • RH <50% • Nonwoven filters for heating and air conditioners • Two-layered "paper" bag for vacuum cleaners
Cat (Fel d 1) and dog (Can f 1)	• Dander • Secretions (cat only)	• 30% of particles are <5 µm and can remain airborne	• Eliminate reservoirs • Air filtration • Wash animals *If unable to eliminate reservoir:* • Avoid animals in primary living areas
German cockroach (Bla g 1 and Bla g 2)	• Breeds in cracks, crevices, etc. • Requires water and food source	• Airborne transiently • Particle size not known	• Hygiene: eliminate all food sources • "Obsessively" filling cracks; closing sites for entry and breeding • Bait: boric acid, pyrethroid traps, glue traps

can act as sensitizers in individuals. The main sources of proteins are dander coming off the skin (for cats and dogs) and urine (for rodents and rabbits). Until recently, saliva was thought to be the main source of cat allergen; however, recent studies have established that secretions from skin glands are the major source of allergen.

The allergen in cat dander is described as being "sticky", because the particles adhere to clothing and furniture and can be detected months after the removal of the animal. In homes where a cat is not present, cat allergen can also be detected. It is thought that the allergen can be passively transferred from schools, from offices, or from a cat that lives outdoors. This passive transfer can cause symptoms or sensitization in individuals who do not have a pet at home (7). Cat allergen remains airborne for long periods of time, and even the slightest airflow can increase the amount of airborne allergen. In fact, several studies have shown that HEPA filters work best in the removal of cat allergen when combined with the removal of carpets and cleaning.

Cat-allergic individuals should be advised to avoid cats even if they do not own one. Cat owners who discover they are cat allergic should be advised to remove the cat from their homes. Another option is to keep the cat outside as much as possible and to wash after handling it. If this is not possible, the individual must control all the sites where the cat allergen accumulates as well as address the source itself. The allergen in dog dander is similar to cat, with smaller particles remaining airborne and being passively transferred from one environment to another.

It can be very difficult to wash a cat that is not accustomed to it. Cats produce large amounts of allergen, and it has been established that the primary source comes from glands in the skin. In theory, washing a cat will remove allergen that would otherwise accumulate in the house. However, studies have shown that washing cats (and even dogs) removes allergens for only a few days, thereby necessitating weekly washing. If this is not practical, wiping pets with a wet washcloth may provide an easier method of removing allergen, albeit one that is not as effective. Keeping a cat restricted to one portion of the house is ineffective, because the allergen is easily transferred around the house. Despite the difficulties, however, some patients are successful in controlling cat allergen exposure in their homes.

German Cockroach

Belying its name, the German cockroach is tropical in origin. It is very difficult for cockroaches to survive outside a residence when temperatures are less than 50°F.

Because cockroaches are more common in multiple-family dwellings than in single-family homes, the German cockroach is an important allergen encountered by families living in low-income environments. It is difficult to control infestation in apartments for several reasons. First, the heated environment of these buildings provides a suitable temperature for cockroaches to breed. Secondly, the allergen can accumulate in areas that are not readily accessible; therefore a reservoir can often be present on the walls and furniture years after the cockroaches have been eradicated. Thirdly, cockroaches are able to hide and breed in many environments; thus it is difficult to effectively spray insecticide in all the infested areas. Cockroaches usually track around the corners of a room, making many commercial bait traps ineffective because they do not fit into these high traffic areas. Spraying large quantities of toxic irritants in the homes of allergic patients also seems counterproductive because this can further exacerbate their symptoms. Lastly, roaches rapidly develop resistance to chemicals that are used in homes.

It is recommended that a professional exterminator apply bait in the home, focusing on corners, in cracks, under furniture, and so on. Newer insecticides, including fipronil, abamectin, and hydromethylnon (8), should be applied. Other methods of controlling these insects include the use of boric acid, "obsessional" caulking to reduce sites of entry where cockroaches can hide and breed, and the use of newer roach traps. Bait traps have been redesigned with a better shape to sit along the wall, a pheromone to attract the roaches, and strong glue in the center surrounded by plastic, which prevents any traction by the roach's legs.

Studies have looked at lifestyle, race, genetics, and quantity of exposure to better understand cockroach allergy. It appears that lifestyle and living conditions in impoverished homes contribute to the sensitization seen in children living in American cities as reported by the National Cooperative Inner City Asthma Study (9). This report cites dryness in apartments in the North and Northeast as greatly inhibiting the growth of dust mites. Most of these apartments do not allow pets so that cat allergen levels are very low in these homes and thus are not a significant cause for sensitization. However, cats also eat cockroaches and could conceivably help prevent accumulation of cockroach allergen in these homes. Furthermore, as mentioned previously, the heated environment of these apartments provides a suitable temperature for cockroach multiplication. If these households, due to the stress of poverty, are not kept clean, cockroaches will easily infest and thrive. Again, the key is to encourage good housekeeping and to eliminate the food and water sources of the cockroach.

In summary, every effort should be made to control the presence of allergen in an allergic patient's environment, even if it means moving to a new home (Case 5-2).

Inner-City Asthma

Recent statistics reveal an alarming rise in inner-city asthma. Living in cities can result in high or low allergen exposure depending on the particular environment. The major situations that can affect clinical outcomes include living in multiple-family dwellings or living in a low-income environment.

Multiple-family dwellings are usually built closer together and higher, which in general can cause a decrease in RH and thereby decrease dust mite growth. Of course, in very humid climates, such as the southern United States, the humidity is higher and growing conditions are always optimal for mites. Rodents and insects readily multiply and travel with ease within multiple-family dwellings. Mice and rats can easily infest a multiple-family dwelling and find nesting sites throughout the building. It is imperative that waste is not stored in the building, and every attempt should be made to keep food encased or refrigerated. If this is not done in the entire building, heavily infested areas can provide a breeding ground for re-infestation despite the best efforts of individual residents.

CASE 5-2   *Patient exposed to an overwhelming quantity of allergens in the home, necessitating a move to a new environment*

A 35-year-old male cardiologist presents with worsening exercise-induced asthma. He has been a distance runner for many years, but over the last year he has been unable to run or even walk without wheezing. He has been compliant with his medications, which include albuterol MDI 2 puffs prn and before exercise, as well as beclomethasone 42 µg/inhalation 2 puffs twice a day. His environmental history reveals that his wheezing developed approximately 6 months after he moved into a basement apartment with carpeting.

His physical examination was normal, with no wheezing on auscultation in any lung field. Skin testing was positive for dust mites. Examination of dust from the carpet revealed the presence of dust mites and a high mite allergen concentration (>10 µg Der p 1/g).

After discussion with the patient and his wife, they decided to move to a second-floor apartment with polished wooden floors. Within 2 months his symptoms had improved, and he had started running again.

Discussion

Basement apartments may be the most difficult environments for allergic patients because they contain large quantities of mite and mold allergens. Some studies have shown that second-floor apartments have a ten-fold less allergen concentration than homes within the same town. Occasionally, moving to a new apartment may be more effective than any other avoidance measures.

Seasonal Inhalants

Although indoor allergens are the focus of this chapter, one should not ignore avoidance of seasonal outdoor allergens. Patients with a hypersensitivity to pollens or mold should be advised to minimize their exposure (e.g., the use of air-conditioning in both homes and cars during peak pollen/mold season). Patients should avoid riding with car windows open or participating in outdoor activities that would increase their exposure (e.g., hay rides, working in a barn). When the patient is working in the yard, particularly when mowing the lawn, a well-fitted facemask can reduce exposure.

Conclusions

Controlling environmental allergen exposure is a realistic goal in the homes of allergic patients. Its success lies in the identification of the exact allergen that is contributing to their symptoms, which can best be accomplished by skin testing or specific serum IgE measurements. Once the association is made, patients often become enthusiastic about modifying their environment.

Enough cannot be said about the importance of educating patients about the specific methods of controlling allergen exposure and supplying them with further reading. The cost of each modification should be outlined so that an individual can make decisions that are both practicable and financially feasible.

In some cases, exposure is so overwhelming that it is not unreasonable to consider moving out of that particular environment into a new home. In addition, patients (particularly students) should be advised about the requirements of a new home if they move.

Criteria for allergen avoidance should not be rigid. Patients should be allowed to make modifications that work for their lifestyle and should be made to feel that they have control over the situation. Often, they will recognize that further modifications are necessary and work hard to make them successful.

■   ■   ■

Key Points

- Dust mites proliferate in humid environments, particularly in clothing, drapes, bedding, and carpets. These allergens can be minimized in the environment through the use of mattress cases and dehumidifiers and by washing linens at high temperatures and eliminating carpets from the home.

- Allergens in cat dander remain airborne for long periods of time. Allergen is best minimized by removing the cat from the home. If that is not possible, the cat should be washed weekly and restricted to nonprimary living areas, and an HEPA filter should be used.

- HEPA filters work best in removing cat allergens from the home when combined with removal of carpets and cleaning.

- Exposure to the cockroach allergen is common in low-income environments. Infestation is best controlled by "obsessional" caulking to reduce sites of entry into the home, diligent housecleaning, and use of some of the newer insecticides and bait traps.

■   ■   ■

REFERENCES

1. **Platts-Mills TA, Tovey ER, Mitchell EB, et al.** Reduction of bronchial hyperreactivity during prolonged allergen avoidance. Lancet. 1982;2:675–8.
2. **Ehnert B, Lau-Schadendort S, Weber A, et al.** Reducing domestic exposure to dust mite allergen reduces bronchial hyperreactivity in sensitive children with asthma. J Allergy Clin Immunol, 1992;90:135–8.

3. **Htut T, Higgenbottom TW, Gill GW, et al.** Eradication of house dust mite from homes of atopic asthmatic subjects: a double-blind trial. J Allergy Clin Immunol, 2001;107:55–60.

4. **Vaughan JW, McLaughlin TE, Perzanowski MS, et al.** Evaluation of materials used for bedding encasement: effect of pore size in blocking cat and dust mite allergen. J Allergy Clin Immunol. 1999;103: 227–31.

5. **Arlian LG, Neal JS, Morgan MS, et al.** Reducing relative humidity is a practical way to control dust mites and their allergens in homes in temperate climates. J Allergy Clin Immunol, 2001;107:99–104.

6. **Platts-Mills TA, Vaughan JW, Carter MC, et al.** The role of intervention in established allergy: avoidance of indoor allergens in the treatment of chronic allergic disease. J Allergy Clin Immunol. 2000;106:787–804.

7. **Almqvist C, Larsson PH, Egmar AC, et al.** School as a risk environment for children allergic to cats and a site for transfer of cat allergen to homes. J Allergy Clin Immunol. 1999;103:1012–7.

8. **Eggleston PA, Arruda LK.** Ecology and elimination of cockroaches and allergens in the home. J Allergy Clin Immunol. 2001;107(3 suppl):S422–9.

9. **Rosenstreich DL, Eggleston P, Kattan M, et al.** The role of cockroach allergy and exposure to cockroach allergen in causing morbidity among inner-city children with asthma. N Engl J Med, 1997;336:1356–63.

6

■   ■   ■

Pharmacotherapy of Asthma

James T. Li, MD

Asthma medications are an important component of the overall management plan for virtually all patients with asthma. The publication *Guidelines for the Diagnosis and Management of Asthma,* published by the National Institutes of Health (NIH), presents a useful scheme for the classification of asthma severity (mild intermittent, mild persistent, moderate persistent, and severe persistent). These guidelines also recommend a stepwise approach to managing asthma with medications (1).

This chapter uses the NIH classification of asthma severity and recommends therapeutic approaches based on this classification (Table 6-1). (The management of acute asthma is discussed in Chapter 4.) Important medications for asthma are reviewed along with recommendations on how and when to use them. This chapter presumes that the diagnosis of asthma is correct, that asthma triggers have been identified and managed, and that the severity of asthma has been properly assessed.

Principles of Pharmacotherapy

The goals of pharmacotherapy of asthma are to control asthma symptoms, improve quality of life, prevent (and treat) asthma exacerbations, and improve lung function, all using the safest and the least amount of medications necessary to reach these goals. Thus prescribing physicians should be familiar with the benefits, risks, and usefulness of each particular asthma medication.

Medications for asthma can be separated into two major categories: medications for as-needed use (termed *quick-relief* medications in the *Guidelines*) and medications for daily use (termed *long-term control* medications in the *Guidelines*). All patients with asthma should have a short-acting

---

Table 6-1   Pharmacotherapy of Asthma by Classification of Severity

Mild Intermittent Asthma

Short-acting beta-agonist as needed for symptoms and for prophylaxis of exercise or allergen-induced asthma

(Second-line: ipratropium or ipratropium/albuterol for as-needed use)

(Second-line: salmeterol, formoterol, nedocromil, cromolyn for prophylaxis)

Mild Persistent Asthma*

Inhaled corticosteroid (low dose)

(Second-line: leukotriene modifier, theophylline, nedocromil)

Moderate Persistent Asthma*

Inhaled corticosteroid (titrate to lowest effective dose

Or

Inhaled corticosteroid in combination with inhaled long-acting beta-agonist

(Consider inhaled corticosteroid plus leukotriene modifier or theophylline)

Severe Persistent Asthma*

Inhaled corticosteroid (titrate to lowest effective dose) *in combination with long-acting inhaled beta-agonist*

(Consider inhaled corticosteroid plus leukotriene modifier or theophylline)

(Consider inhaled corticosteroid plus inhaled long-acting beta-agonist plus leukotriene modifier)

Or

Inhaled corticosteroid (titrate to lowest effective dose)

(If asthma is not well controlled, add oral corticosteroids)

---

* Patients with persistent asthma should use a short-acting bronchodilator for as-needed and prophylactic use.

bronchodilator (e.g., albuterol metered dose inhaler [MDI]) for as-needed use. Patients classified as having persistent asthma (mild, moderate, or severe persistent asthma) should be using at least one daily (long-term controller) asthma medication.

Asthma medications are administered orally or by inhalation. Commonly prescribed oral asthma medications include the leukotriene modifiers and theophylline. Oral beta-agonists are available (but not generally recommended), and oral corticosteroids are used in select patients with severe, corticosteroid-dependent asthma. Asthma medications administered by inhalation can be delivered by a variety of inhalation delivery devices including MDIs, dry powder inhalers (DPIs), and nebulizers. Metered dose inhalers use either CFC (chlorofluorocarbons) propellants or non-CFC propellants such as HFA (hydrofluoroalkane), can be breath-actuated (or not), and can be used with spacer devices (or not). Most patients require careful and repeated instruction and coaching in order to use inhaler devices properly. Nebulizers are inefficient delivery devices and generally are not recommended for home use for most patients. Aerosol delivery by nebulization is recommended for the treatment of acute asthma.

Medications

Short-Acting Beta-Agonists

Products
Short-acting beta-agonists are usually prescribed as MDIs. Albuterol is available as a generic product, as a branded CFC MDI (Ventolin), and as a non-CFC MDI (Proventil-HFA). Generic albuterol is as effective as branded albuterol. Pirbuterol is available as a breath-actuated MDI (Maxair Autohaler). Albuterol delivered by single-dose DPI (Ventolin Rotacaps) is less convenient than MDIs for most patients. Racemic albuterol delivered by nebulization is the first-line treatment for acute asthma but should be used infrequently for chronic asthma.

Mechanisms
Albuterol, levalbuterol, and pirbuterol are selective beta-2 agonists that act as bronchodilators. These agents are only partially beta-2 selective, and beta-2 receptors are found in the heart as well as the lung. Thus beta-2 agonists can cause unwanted sympathomimetic effects such as tachycardia, palpitations, and tremor.

Beta-agonists bind to beta-2 receptors in the lung that activate G proteins and adenyl cyclase in smooth muscle cells, leading to activation of protein kinase A and relaxation of bronchial smooth muscle. Beta-agonists are effective bronchodilators. The onset of bronchodilatation occurs within minutes of inhalation, peaks at about 15 min, and has a maximum duration of action of about 5 to 8 hr.

Indications
Inhaled short-acting beta-agonists are indicated for the as-needed control of asthma symptoms. This is often described as "rescue" or "quick-relief" therapy. Inhaled short-acting beta-agonists are indicated for prophylaxis of exercise-induced asthma and asthma provoked by allergen triggers (Case 6-1).

Safety
Short-acting beta-agonists may cause unwanted effects such as tremor, increased heart rate, or headache. Beta-agonists may cause hypokalemia, hyperglycemia, and prolongation of the corrected QT interval, although these effects are usually not clinically significant. Paradoxical bronchospasm may develop in some patients. This can usually be managed by changing canisters or switching to a different product.

CASE 6-1   *Patient with mild intermittent asthma*

An 18-year-old man presents with episodic shortness of breath. Symptoms of shortness of breath and wheezing developed at age 6 years but have been mild. He reports a few occasions of increased wheezing with the common cold, but these symptoms usually resolve in 1 to 2 weeks without treatment. The patient reports chest tightness and shortness of breath when playing outdoor full-court basketball in the summer, but not with other sports. Symptoms may also be triggered when he shovels snow, and when he visits his grandmother who has a cat. On average, he experiences some respiratory symptoms 3 or 4 times a month. He has used a friend's inhaler with good symptomatic relief.

Physical examination is unremarkable. Spirometry shows a baseline FEV_1 of 93% predicted, which increases by 4% after inhaled albuterol.

Discussion

The clinical presentation strongly suggests mild intermittent asthma. Clinically relevant triggers for this patient are exercise, cold air, allergens, and respiratory infections. The pharmacologic treatment for this patient should include a short-acting bronchodilator (e.g., albuterol MDI, pirbuterol MDI) for use as-needed for quick relief and for use before exercise and before cat exposure.

Ipratropium may be considered as a second-line quick-relief bronchodilator, but nothing in this patient's presentation suggests that ipratropium is a good choice for him. Likewise, salmeterol, nedocromil, or cromolyn may be considered as second-line agents for exercise and allergen prophylaxis, but they are not the best choices for this patient at this time.

Overuse of inhaled beta-agonists has been linked to fatal and near-fatal asthma. Most experts believe that the increased use of short-acting beta-agonists in the setting of acute undertreated asthma is what accounts for this association; in other words, the high use of beta-agonists in fatal asthma is a marker for severe acute undertreated asthma, rather than a cause of it. Some studies have shown that the regular, continuous use of short-acting beta-agonists can result in a small increase in bronchial hyper-responsiveness. However, clinical studies show that regularly scheduled short-acting beta-agonists are equally as effective (and no worse than) on-demand beta-agonists (2).

Recommendations

Inhaled short-acting bronchodilators are recommended for as-needed use (quick relief) for asthma symptoms, for prophylaxis of exercise-induced asthma, and for prophylaxis of allergen-induced asthma. All patients with asthma should have a short-acting bronchodilator for as-needed use. Patients with mild intermittent asthma usually need no other asthma medication than a short-acting bronchodilator. The usual dose of albuterol MDI or pirbuterol MDI is 2 puffs 4 times daily as needed. Some patients achieve effective bronchodilatation with 1 puff.

As with all inhalation devices, patients using inhaled short-acting beta-agonists should receive repeated instruction and coaching on the proper use of the delivery device (usually an MDI for short-acting beta-agonists such as albuterol or pirbuterol). A spacer device can be helpful for patients with suboptimal hand-lung coordination, but it is not necessary for all patients. It is also not necessary to precede inhalation of inhaled corticosteroids (or nedocromil or cromolyn) with short-acting beta-agonists.

Assessment of as-needed bronchodilator use is a good measure of asthma control. Patients whose asthma is well controlled use little as-needed bronchodilator, whereas patients with poorly controlled asthma or with an asthma exacerbation may use short-acting bronchodilators several times a day (or night). High use of as-needed bronchodilators (3 or 4 times a day or 1 or 2 cannisters a month) should alert the physician that asthma may be poorly controlled.

Ipratropium

Products
Ipratropium bromide (Atrovent) is available as an MDI and as a solution for nebulization. Ipratropium combined with albuterol (Combivent) is available in MDI form.

Mechanisms
Ipratropium is an anticholinergic agent administered by inhalation. Anticholinergic agents block muscarinic receptors that regulate airway tone and mucus production. Ipratropium is a short-acting bronchodilator. Bronchodilation peaks around 1 to 2 hr after inhalation and persists for about 3 to 4 hr.

Indications
Ipratropium does not carry an approved indication for use in asthma. However, ipratropium may be a useful alternative for people who are intolerant to the side effects of inhaled albuterol. Ipratropium with albuterol by nebulization has been used for treatment of acute bronchospasm.

Safety
Ipratropium is well tolerated by most patients. Ipratropium MDI causes occasional cough and dry mouth.

Recommendations
Ipratropium is a first-line bronchodilator for use in chronic obstructive pulmonary disease. In asthma, ipratropium MDI can be used as a second-line

short-acting bronchodilator for as-needed (or quick relief) use. The short-acting beta-agonists are preferred for as-needed (or quick relief) use in asthma. Ipratropium by nebulization (in combination with nebulized albuterol) may have a role in acute asthma but is not indicated for the treatment of chronic asthma. The combination of ipratropium and albuterol MDI can be considered for as-needed (quick relief) use in asthma, but studies supporting this indication are lacking.

Long-Acting Beta-Agonists

Products
Salmeterol (Serevent) (3) and formoterol (Foradil) (4) are inhaled long-acting beta-agonists. Salmeterol is available in MDI and DPI formulations. Formoterol is available as a DPI. Albuterol is available as a sustained-release oral formulation. Fluticasone and salmeterol combined in a single-delivery device (Advair) is available.

Mechanisms
Long-acting beta-agonists have extended hydrophobic side chains. The lipophilic side chains of the molecule may interact with the lipid bilayer of the cell membrane, leading to a prolonged duration of action. Other studies suggest that long-acting beta-agonists may bind to the beta-2 receptor at a domain other than the active site, thus leading to a prolonged duration of action.

Bronchodilation begins approximately 10 min following an inhalation of salmeterol, and peak response is reached after several hours. Bronchodilation begins in only 3 min following an inhalation of formoterol, with peak bronchodilation in about 1 hr. Both salmeterol and formoterol have a duration of action of approximately 12 hr.

Indications
Inhaled long-acting beta-agonists are used twice daily in combination with inhaled corticosteroids in the treatment of moderate persistent or severe persistent asthma. Inhaled long-acting beta-agonists are indicated for prophylaxis of exercise-induced asthma, especially if prolonged exercise is anticipated. Inhaled long-acting beta-agonists in the evening are effective in the treatment of nocturnal asthma.

Safety
The adverse effects of long-acting beta-agonists are similar to the adverse effects of short-acting bronchodilators (tremor, increased heart rate, hyperglycemia, hypokalemia). Continuous use of salmeterol can result in a diminution of the bronchoprotective effect of salmeterol (against exercise or bronchial challenge). However, continuous use of salmeterol does not result in a reduction of bronchodilatation.

Recommendations

The combination of inhaled long-acting beta-agonists and an inhaled corticosteroid is highly effective in the treatment of moderate and severe persistent asthma. Comparison studies show that this combination is superior to inhaled corticosteroids alone, even at high doses. For moderately severe persistent asthma, inhaled long-acting beta-agonists can be added to inhaled corticosteroids, especially if the asthma is not well controlled on a low or medium dose of inhaled corticosteroids. The combination of inhaled long-acting beta-agonists and inhaled corticosteroids should be considered the treatment of choice for severe asthma. This combination can be delivered by using two different inhalers, or with the fluticasone/salmeterol combination product (5).

Inhaled long-acting beta-agonists are effective in the treatment of nocturnal asthma. Sustained-release albuterol and sustained-release theophylline are two other agents with demonstrated efficacy in treating nocturnal asthma. Inhaled long-acting beta-agonists are generally preferred for this indication because of superior efficacy and favorable adverse effect profile.

Inhaled long-acting beta-agonists are effective for prophylaxis of exercise-induced asthma. However, as already mentioned, continuous use of inhaled long-acting beta-agonists can lead to a diminished protective effect against exercise. For this reason, short-acting beta-agonists are the first-line choice for exercise-induced asthma.

Inhaled long-acting beta-agonists should not be used for rescue or quick relief of asthma symptoms. Inhaled long-acting beta-agonists should not be used as a single agent because these agents exert little, if any, antiinflammatory effect. Inhaled long-acting beta-agonists should not be used in mild intermittent or mild persistent asthma. The recommended dose of inhaled long-acting beta-agonists is 2 puffs 2 times a day for salmeterol MDI and one puff twice a day for salmeterol or formoterol DPI.

Inhaled Corticosteroids

Products

Several inhaled corticosteroid products are available (Table 6-2). There are specific drug moieties (beclomethasone, budesonide, flunisolide, fluticasone, triamcinolone), different delivery devices (MDI, DPI), different MDI propellants (CFC, HFA), and combination products (fluticasone/salmeterol).

Mechanisms

Corticosteroids have broad antiinflammatory effects in asthma. Through modulation of transcription factors, corticosteroids inhibit the production of inflammatory cytokines such as IL4 and IL5. Studies involving bronchial biopsies in patients with asthma show that inhaled corticosteroids reduce local cytokine production, reduce inflammatory cell infiltration of airway mucosa, and improve bronchial hyperresponsiveness.

Table 6-2   Estimated Comparative Daily Dosages for Inhaled Corticosteroids

Drug	Trade Name	Low Dose	Medium Dose	High Dose
Beclomethasone dipropionate	Vanceril, Beclovent	168-504 µg	504-840 µg	>840 µg
CFC-MDI: 42 µg/puff		(4-12 puffs– 42 µg)	(12-20 puffs– 42 µg)	
CFC-MDI: 84 µg/puff		(2-6 puffs– 84 µg)	(6-10 puffs– 84 µg)	(>10 puffs– 84 µg)
Beclomethasone dipropionate	QVAR	80-160 µg	160-320 µg	>320 µg
HFA-MDI: 40 µg/puff		(2-4 puffs– 40 µg)	(4-8 puffs– 40 µg)	(>8 puffs– 40 µg)
HFA-MDI: 80 µg/puff		(1-2 puffs– 80 µg)	(2-4 puffs– 80 µg)	(>4 puffs– 80 µg)
Budesonide	Pulmicort	200-400 µg	400-600 µg	>600 µg
DPI: 200 µg/dose		(1-2 inhalations)	(2-3 inhalations)	(>3 inhalations)
Flunisolide	Aerobid	500-1000 µg	1000-2000 µg	>2000 µg
MDI: 250 µg/puff		(2-4 puffs)	(4-8 puffs)	(>8 puffs)
Fluticasone	Flovent	88-264 µg	264-660 µg	>660 µg
MDI: 44, 110, 220 µg/puff		(2-6 puffs– 44 µg) or (2 puffs– 110 µg)	(2-6 puffs– 110 µg)	(>6 puffs– 110 µg) or (>3 puffs– 200 µg)
DPI: 50, 100, 250 µg/dose		(2-6 inhalations– 50 µg)	(3-6 inhalations– 100 µg)	(>6 inhalations– 100 µg) or (>2 inhalations– 220 µg)
Triamcinolone acetonide	Azmacort	400-1000 µg	1000-2000 µg	>2000 µg
MDI: 100 µg/puff		(4-10 puffs)	(10-20 puffs)	(>20 puffs)

Modified from Guidelines for the Diagnosis and Management of Asthma. NIH Publication 98-4051;1998:88.

Inhaled corticosteroids are highly effective in the treatment of chronic asthma. Inhaled corticosteroids have been shown to reduce asthma symptoms, supplemental bronchodilator use, asthma exacerbations, and asthma mortality.

Indications
Inhaled corticosteroids are indicated in the treatment of mild, moderate, and severe persistent asthma. Inhaled corticosteroids should be considered first-line treatment for all patients with persistent asthma.

Safety

Inhaled corticosteroids may cause local adverse effects such as dysphonia and oral candidiasis. These local effects may occur in about 20% of patients. Using a spacer device that reduces the oropharyngeal deposition of corticosteroid can reduce the frequency of oral candidiasis. Oral antifungal agents may be necessary to treat episodes of candidiasis.

Inhaled corticosteroids are associated with a small dose-dependent risk of systemic corticosteroid side effects (6) (see section on Oral Corticosteroids below). The effect on bone seems to be a very sensitive indicator of the systemic effects of inhaled corticosteroids. Inhaled corticosteroids can reduce growth velocity in children (by about 1 to 1.5 cm) and can decrease bone density in adults. The effect of inhaled corticosteroids on the final adult height of children is not known and may be very small or trivial. Likewise, the risk of osteoporosis and pathologic fractures caused by inhaled corticosteroids is small.

There may be a small increased risk of posterior subcapsular cataracts and increased intraocular pressure in patients using large doses of long-term inhaled corticosteroids. Inhaled corticosteroids can cause a dose-dependent suppression of HPA axis function. This effect does not generally cause symptoms of adrenal insufficiency. Finally, the risk of bruising may be increased with inhaled corticosteroids.

Recommendations

Inhaled corticosteroids are the most effective long-term treatment for asthma, and should be considered first-line therapy for all patients with persistent asthma. As a single agent, inhaled corticosteroids are more effective than theophylline, salmeterol, nedocromil, and leukotriene modifiers. Generally, spacer devices are used with MDIs in order to reduce oropharyngeal deposition.

Most inhaled corticosteroid products can be administered twice a day. Some inhaled corticosteroids can be taken just once a day, which improves adherence. All patients should be carefully instructed and coached on how to use the corticosteroid inhalation device.

DOSE-RESPONSE RELATIONSHIP

At commonly prescribed doses (e.g., 4 to 8 puffs/day), inhaled corticosteroids demonstrate a relatively flat dose-response curve. Typically, the dose of inhaled corticosteroid must be increased two- to ten-fold in order to demonstrate greater efficacy. Furthermore, inhaled corticosteroids may be effective at lower than generally prescribed doses (e.g., 2 puffs/day).

In principle, each patient should use the lowest effective dose required to achieve good control of asthma. Control of asthma should be assessed periodically by evaluation of symptoms, supplemental bronchodilator use, exacerbations, peak flow, and spirometry. The dose of inhaled corticosteroid can be adjusted so that the lowest effective dose is used.

The lowest effective dose of inhaled corticosteroid may be different for different patients. Nevertheless, as a general rule, patients with more severe asthma will require higher doses of inhaled corticosteroid in order to achieve good asthma control.

SELECTION OF SPECIFIC INHALED CORTICOSTEROID PRODUCTS

The two major factors to consider when selecting a corticosteroid are the specific drug and the inhalation delivery device. In fact, the two factors are so closely intertwined that it is best to view each individual inhaled corticosteroid product as a drug/delivery device system. For example, comparative studies suggest that fluticasone MDI is about twice as potent as beclomethasone CFC-MDI. Thus approximately half as much fluticasone MDI can be expected to be as effective as beclomethasone CFC-MDI.

Studies show that the budesonide DPI device can deliver about twice as much medication to the lower airway than a comparable budesonide or beclomethasone CFC-MDI. Beclomethasone HFA-MDI delivers over twice as much medication to the lower airway as beclomethasone CFC-MDI. Thus half the dose of budesonide DPI or beclomethasone HFA-MDI should achieve about the same efficacy as beclomethasone CFC-MDI. Although not completely studied, triamcinolone MDI and flunisolide MDI are equipotent or less potent than beclomethasone CFC-MDI.

Selection of a particular inhaled corticosteroid should involve patient preferences. Some patients may prefer either a MDI or DPI, or the design of a particular inhalation device. Some patients have poor hand-lung coordination skills and may prefer a breath-actuated device (such as a DPI). Spacer devices are often used with MDIs and should be prescribed with patient preference in mind.

High-potency inhaled corticosteroids (e.g., fluticasone) or high-efficiency delivery devices (e.g., budesonide DPI, beclomethasone HFA MDI) should be considered for patients with moderate or severe asthma. These products (particularly fluticasone MDI) may be more *effective* than other inhaled corticosteroids such as beclomethasone CFC-MDI. However, the safety of high-potency inhaled corticosteroids (e.g., fluticasone) or high-efficiency delivery devices (e.g., budesonide DPI, beclomethasone HFA MDI) relative to beclomethasone CFC-MDI has been incompletely studied. For example, fluticasone MDI may have a greater suppressive effect on HPA axis function than beclomethasone CFC MDI but may also have less effect on growth. The effect of beclomethasone HFA MDI on growth in children has not been fully studied.

INHALED CORTICOSTEROIDS COMBINED WITH OTHER ASTHMA MEDICATIONS

The addition of a second long-term asthma medication (inhaled long-acting beta-agonists, leukotriene modifiers, theophylline, and, to a lesser extent, nedocromil) to an inhaled corticosteroid is usually more effective than an inhaled corticosteroid as a single agent. The addition of inhaled long-acting beta-agonists, montelukast, or theophylline to medium-dose inhaled corti-costeroids is more effective than doubling the dose of inhaled cortico-steroids.

A direct comparison study showed that the combination of an inhaled corticosteroid plus salmeterol was more effective than the inhaled cortico-steroid plus montelukast. Although direct comparison studies are lacking, other clinical studies suggest that an inhaled long-acting beta-agonist com-bined with an inhaled corticosteroid is the most effective combination. The addition of a second long-term asthma medication may allow the use of a lower dose of inhaled corticosteroids while maintaining good control of asthma.

A combination fluticasone-salmeterol DPI (Advair) is available in three dose formulations (fluticasone 100 µg, fluticasone 250 µg, and fluticasone 500 µg, each combined with salmeterol 50 µg). This combination inhaler is a convenient way to deliver an inhaled corticosteroid plus a long-acting beta-agonist. The availability of three dose formulations permits the selec-tion of the appropriate dose for patients with moderate persistent and severe persistent asthma. Other corticosteroid/long-acting bronchodilator combination inhalers are in development.

RECOMMENDATIONS FOR MILD, MODERATE, AND SEVERE PERSISTENT ASTHMA
Inhaled corticosteroids at low dose is the first-line treatment for *mild persis-tent asthma* (Case 6-2). This therapy is effective and carries a very low risk of systemic adverse effects. There are other therapeutic options for individ-ual patients, including leukotriene modifiers, theophylline, and nedocromil. Patients who do not tolerate inhaled corticosteroids, who wish to avoid corticosteroids, or who prefer oral agents may be candidates for one of these options.

Patients with *moderate persistent asthma* should use an inhaled corti-costeroid (Case 6-3). The dose of inhaled corticosteroid for these patients should be titrated to the lowest effective dose. The lowest effective dose of inhaled corticosteroid for an individual patient with moderately severe per-sistent asthma may be a low, medium, or high dose. Patients whose asthma is not fully controlled by low or medium dose inhaled corticosteroids should use a combination of inhaled corticosteroid plus an inhaled long-acting beta-agonist, leukotriene modifier, or (if tolerated) theophylline. High-potency inhaled corticosteroids (e.g., fluticasone) or high-efficiency delivery devices (e.g., budesonide DPI, beclomethasone HFA MDI) should be considered for patients with moderate or severe asthma.

All patients with *severe persistent asthma* should use an inhaled cortico-steroid, with the same considerations as described above for patients with moderate persistent asthma (Case 6-4). High-potency inhaled corticosteroids (e.g., fluticasone) may be a good choice for some patients with severe asthma. A trial of inhaled corticosteroid *plus* an inhaled long-acting beta-agonist *plus* a leukotriene modifier (i.e., three medications) is reasonable

---

CASE 6-2   *Patient with mild persistent asthma*

A 35-year-old college professor presents with increasing shortness of breath. He reports episodes of shortness of breath, chest tightness, and occasional wheezing since age 12 years. In the past year, he has experienced these symptoms upon awakening 2 or 3 times a week and at work about 3 or 4 times a week. The patient has an albuterol MDI that he uses 4 or 5 times a week in the spring, summer, and fall, but less often in the winter. He would like more effective asthma treatment but is wary about taking steroids.

Physical examination is unremarkable. Spirometry shows an FEV$_1$ of 89% predicted that increases by 10% after inhaled albuterol.

Discussion

Presentation suggests mild persistent asthma. This patient should be using a daily "long-term" control medication for his asthma; an inhaled corticosteroid is the first-choice and most effective agent in this setting. The expressed concern about steroid side effects should be addressed fully with the patient. The dose-response relationship of inhaled corticosteroids suggests that this patient may achieve excellent control of asthma using low doses (once daily if possible) of inhaled corticosteroids (which carry a very small risk of systemic corticosteroid adverse effects).

Leukotriene modifiers, theophylline, cromolyn, and nedocromil may be options for this patient. These agents are not as effective as inhaled corticosteroids. However, after careful consideration and discussion, the patient may prefer or choose to take a noncorticosteroid asthma medication. The potential side effects and drug-drug interactions of theophylline may limit its use in this patient. The requirement for multiple daily doses with some agents (e.g., cromolyn, zileuton, nedocromil, zafirlukast) or monitoring of liver function with others (e.g., zileuton, zafirlukast) are other considerations. Montelukast may be an option.

---

for patients whose asthma is not well controlled by inhaled corticosteroid plus a long-acting inhaled beta-agonist. Patients with severe asthma that is difficult to control may require continuous oral corticosteroids.

Theophylline

Products

Theophylline is most often prescribed as a sustained-release oral formulation. Some products are formulated for once daily use. Short-acting oral formulations and liquid suspensions are infrequently used in adults. Theophylline preparations are usually less expensive than branded inhalers.

Mechanisms

Theophylline is a bronchodilator, with a small protective effect against exercise or bronchial challenge (7). The mechanism of action of theophylline

---

CASE 6-3   *Patient with moderate persistent asthma*

A 54-year-old woman presents with increasing shortness of breath and wheezing. She reports a 15-year history of asthma that has been worsening over the past year. She experiences shortness of breath with some wheezing almost every day. Current asthma medications are beclomethasone CFC-MDI 4 puffs twice a day and albuterol MDI 2 puffs 3 or 4 times daily. Past asthma history is notable for 3 or 4 hospitalizations and 5 or 6 emergency department visits for asthma over the past 10 years. The most recent emergency department visit for asthma was 6 months ago, and the most recent course of oral corticosteroids was 3 months ago.

Physical examination is unremarkable. There is no respiratory distress and no audible wheezing. Spirometry shows an FEV_1 of 67% predicted with a 12% increase after inhaled albuterol.

Discussion

This patient has moderate persistent asthma according to NIH Guidelines criteria. There are a number of therapeutic considerations and options for this patient.

One strategy is to intensify treatment using an inhaled corticosteroid as a single agent. For example, one could double the dose of inhaled beclomethasone CFC-MDI to 8 puffs twice day. However, compliance may be a problem, and current therapy with this agent has not been effective according to the history. Another option is to change to a different inhaled corticosteroid product, particularly one with greater potency or greater lung deposition. Examples of such products include fluticasone MDI or DPI, budesonide DPI, and beclomethasone HFA-MDI. Medium or high doses may be appropriate with these products for this patient.

Another strategy is to use a combination of inhaled corticosteroids and a second long-term asthma medication. The most effective combination of asthma medications is probably an inhaled corticosteroid plus an inhaled long-acting beta-agonist. Montelukast or zafirlukast plus inhaled corticosteroids have been well studied and may be a suitable choice if inhaled long-acting beta-agonists are not tolerated. Inhaled corticosteroids combined with either theophylline or nedocromil may be considered, but each of these combinations may not be as effective as the other options. High doses of inhaled corticosteroids may not be needed if combined with a long-acting beta-agonist in this patient.

---

in asthma is unclear. Theophylline is a nonselective inhibitor of cAMP phosphodiesterases in airway smooth muscle and inflammatory cells, and is an antagonist of adenosine receptors.

Theophylline inhibits the activation and release of inflammatory mediators from eosinophils and T cells *in vitro*. Theophylline has been shown to reduce eosinophil recruitment and the late-phase asthmatic response induced by allergen challenge. However, the overall importance of these anti-inflammatory effects of theophylline is small.

CASE 6-4   *Patient with severe persistent asthma*

A 39-year-old man presents for evaluation of asthma. He presents to the clinic (at the insistence of his wife) following a severe asthma exacerbation. A year before presentation he experienced a severe asthma attack, one not responsive to inhaled albuterol. This asthma exacerbation resulted in a respiratory arrest, intubation, and intensive care unit admission. Since that time he has been using an inhaled corticosteroid and inhaled salmeterol. He uses albuterol MDI 5 or 6 times daily for symptoms of shortness of breath. Over the past year he has required three courses of oral corticosteroids but no further hospitalizations.

Physical examination reveals a prolonged expiratory phase and end-expiratory wheezes. Spirometry shows a baseline FEV_1 of 45% predicted with a 17% increase after inhaled albuterol.

Discussion

This patient has severe persistent asthma according to NIH Guidelines criteria. His asthma medications should include a high-dose, high-potency inhaled corticosteroid administered through an efficient delivery device (e.g., fluticasone MDI 440 µg twice a day or budesonide DPI 800 µg twice a day) plus a long-acting beta-agonist. One might consider adding a leukotriene modifier to the combination of inhaled corticosteroids plus inhaled long-acting beta-agonist.

A critical decision for this patient is whether to begin daily or alternate-day corticosteroids. A therapeutic trial of daily or alternate-day corticosteroids may be appropriate while continuing to monitor symptoms, albuterol use, home peak flow rates, and office spirometry.

Indications

Theophylline is a second- or third-line agent for the daily treatment of persistent asthma. Theophylline can be used as a single agent in mild asthma but should be considered a second agent because of its relatively unfavorable adverse effect profile. Sustained-release theophylline is effective in nocturnal asthma, although inhaled long-acting beta-agonists may be preferred for most patients. For moderate or severe asthma, theophylline can be combined with an inhaled corticosteroid.

Safety

The adverse effects of theophylline include nausea, headache, insomnia, diarrhea, irritability, tremors, and diuresis. Adverse effects at higher doses (or higher serum theophylline concentrations) include vomiting, cardiac arrhythmias, and seizures. Many medications interfere with the cytochrome p450 metabolism of theophylline. Medications that can decrease the clearance of theophylline (hence can increase theophylline levels) include macrolide antibiotics, ciprofloxacin, propranolol, diltiazem, verapamil, disulfiram, and oral contraceptives. Medications that can increase theophylline clearance (hence can decrease theophylline levels) include phenytoin, phenobarbital, and cimetidine).

Recommendations

Theophylline is an effective medication for asthma, but its use is limited by the high frequency of adverse effects and its drug-drug interactions. Patients taking theophylline should have periodic measurements of serum theophylline concentrations in order to reduce the risk of theophylline toxicity. The recommended therapeutic range is 5 to15 µg/mL. Studies comparing theophylline to other asthma treatments show that theophylline is not as effective as inhaled corticosteroids when used as a single agent for mild-to-moderate asthma. Salmeterol was superior to theophylline in the treatment of nocturnal asthma.

Theophylline (as a single agent) can be considered for patients with mild persistent asthma who are unable or unwilling to use inhaled corticosteroids. Some patients are unable to use inhalation devices (even after careful instruction) or greatly prefer oral agents. Growing children with mild persistent asthma may prefer to avoid using an agent (inhaled corticosteroids) that can inhibit growth. Some patients tolerate theophylline well, without adverse effects. Low doses of theophylline (with serum theophylline concentrations of 5 to 10 µg/mL) are usually better tolerated than higher doses.

Patients with moderate persistent (or severe persistent) asthma often need therapy with more than one medication. Studies show that the combination of theophylline with an inhaled corticosteroid is more effective than an inhaled corticosteroid alone, even at high doses. However, many asthma experts prefer the combination of inhaled long-acting beta-agonists with inhaled corticosteroids for patients who need more than inhaled corticosteroids alone.

Leukotriene Modifiers

Products

The leukotriene modifying agents are all orally administered. Zileuton (Zyflo) is a lipoxygenase inhibitor that is usually prescribed for use four times a day. Zafirlukast (Accolate) and montelukast (Singulair) are leukotriene receptor antagonists. Zafirlukast is usually taken twice a day and montelukast is usually taken once a day.

Mechanisms

Leukotrienes are inflammatory mediators that are products of arachidonic metabolism (8). The leukotrienes play a role in inflammation and bronchospasm in asthma. The five lipoxygenase inhibitors (e.g., zileuton) inhibit the formation of leukotrienes (LTB4, LTC4, LTD4, and LTE4). The leukotriene receptor antagonists (e.g., zafirlukast, montelukast) inhibit the binding of cysteinyl leukotrienes (LTC4, LTD4, and LTE4) to the cysteinyl leukotriene receptor.

Indications

The leukotriene modifiers are indicated for the treatment of persistent asthma. A leukotriene modifier can be used as a single agent for mild persistent asthma. Montelukast and zafirlukast can be used in combination with an inhaled corticosteroid for moderate or severe persistent asthma.

Safety

Zileuton and zafirlukast may cause elevation of liver function tests. These two agents have been associated with rare instances of severe liver injury. The leukotriene modifiers have been linked to cases of Churg-Strauss vasculitis. Some observers have suggested that these cases may have had a primary eosinophilic disorder that was unmasked as corticosteroids were withdrawn. However, eosinophilic infiltrative disorders have been associated with leukotriene modifier use even in the absence of previous corticosteroid therapy.

Zafirlukast can interfere with warfarin therapy.

Recommendations

The leukotriene modifiers are appropriate for use as single agents in mild persistent asthma. These agents are effective in the treatment of chronic asthma and exercise induced asthma. The four times daily dosing requirement, the risk of hepatic injury, and the need to monitor liver function tests limit the usefulness of zileuton (and to a lesser extent zafirlukast). Comparative studies suggest that the leukotriene modifiers are about as effective as theophylline or cromolyn but not as effective as inhaled corticosteroids. The leukotriene modifiers should be considered for patients with mild persistent asthma who prefer an oral agent or who are unable or unwilling to use corticosteroids. Growing children with mild persistent asthma may prefer to avoid using an agent (inhaled corticosteroids) that can inhibit growth.

The generation of leukotrienes is thought to play an important role in the development of aspirin-induced asthma. Indeed, the leukotriene modifiers are effective in treating asthma in aspirin-sensitive patients. However, patients who are highly sensitive to aspirin may develop severe bronchospasm after aspirin ingestion, even when pretreated with leukotriene modifying agents.

Studies show that the combination of montelukast or zafirlukast with an inhaled corticosteroid is more effective than inhaled corticosteroids alone. This combination is appropriate for patients with moderate or severe persistent asthma. A comparative trial showed that the combination of salmeterol and an inhaled corticosteroid was more effective than the combination of montelukast and an inhaled corticosteroid. Thus the combination of salmeterol and inhaled corticosteroids is preferred over the combination of montelukast or zafirlukast and inhaled corticosteroids for most patients. The triple combination of inhaled corticosteroids, salmeterol, and a leukotriene modifier can be considered for patients with severe asthma; however, this therapy has not been adequately studied.

The leukotriene modifiers are effective in reducing symptoms of allergic rhinitis. This may be a consideration for patients with coexisting asthma and allergic rhinitis.

Nedocromil and Cromolyn

Products
Nedocromil is available as an MDI. Cromolyn is available as an MDI, DPI, and as a solution for nebulization. The MDI formulation is preferred for adults.

Mechanisms
The mechanisms by which nedocromil and cromolyn are effective in asthma are unknown. It is known that these compounds inhibit mast cell mediator release *in vitro,* inhibit the early- and late-phase asthmatic responses to inhaled allergen challenge, and are bronchoprotective for exercise. Continuous treatment with nedocromil or cromolyn can reduce bronchial hyperreactivity.

Indications
Nedocromil and cromolyn are second-line agents that may be used in mild persistent asthma. Both are second-line agents that can be used for prophylaxis of exercise-induced asthma and allergen-induced asthma.

Safety
Nedocromil and cromolyn have very few significant side effects. About 20% of patients find the taste of nedocromil unpleasant.

Recommendations
Comparative studies show that nedocromil and cromolyn are equally effective in adults, although nedocromil may be more effective than cromolyn in children. Both products are about as effective as leukotriene modifiers and theophylline. Neither product is as effective as inhaled corticosteroids. Nedocromil and cromolyn can be considered for patients with mild persistent asthma who are unwilling or unable to take inhaled corticosteroids or who are concerned about corticosteroid side effects. The usual dosing for both products is 2 puffs 4 times a day, although some studies show that nedocromil can be given twice a day.

Nedocromil and cromolyn can be used for prophylaxis of exercise-induced asthma or before an anticipated allergen exposure. Short-acting beta-agonists are the preferred prophylactic agents for these indications, but nedocromil or cromolyn may be considered if short-acting beta-agonists are not fully effective. Furthermore, beta-agonists can be combined with nedocromil or cromolyn for prophylaxis of exercise or allergen-induced asthma, although studies demonstrating an additive effect are lacking.

Some studies suggest that there may be an additive effect in adding nedocromil (but not cromolyn) to inhaled corticosteroids. However, this additive effect is small and inconsistent. Nedocromil and cromolyn are not recommended for moderate or severe persistent asthma.

Oral Corticosteroids

Products
Many oral corticosteroid products are available. Prednisone is the best studied and least expensive oral corticosteroid product commonly used in asthma.

Mechanisms
As with inhaled corticosteroids, oral corticosteroids have broad anti-inflammatory effects in asthma (see section on Inhaled Corticosteroids above). Corticosteroids reduce mucosal edema, mucus production, and airway inflammation in asthma.

Indications
Systemic corticosteroids are indicated for the treatment of acute asthma (see Chapter 4) and for the patient with severe persistent asthma whose asthma is not well controlled by inhaled corticosteroids and other agents.

Safety
The adverse effects of systemic corticosteroids include hyperglycemia, electrolyte disturbances, growth suppression, osteoporosis, posterior subcapsular cataracts, fat redistribution, bruising, mood disorders, increased susceptibility to infection, and HPA axis suppression.

Recommendations
Oral corticosteroids are indicated for the outpatient treatment of acute asthma or poorly controlled asthma. Some patients have severe persistent asthma that is not well controlled by the combination of inhaled corticosteroids and a second (or third) long-term asthma medication. These patients with severe persistent asthma may require continuous oral corticosteroids.

The dose of continuous oral corticosteroid should be titrated to the "lowest effective dose." Control of asthma should be assessed periodically by evaluation of symptoms, supplemental bronchodilator use, exacerbations, peak flow, and spirometry. The dose of oral corticosteroid can be adjusted so that the lowest effective dose is used.

Continuous oral corticosteroids can be administered daily or on alternate days. The alternate-day regimen may reduce systemic adverse effects to a limited extent. Patients on continuous corticosteroid therapy usually take a dose once a day in the morning. A study suggested that a single dose of oral corticosteroid taken in the afternoon was more effective than a single dose in the morning. There may be less HPA axis suppression with the afternoon dosing schedule. However, the morning dose schedule more closely mimics the physiologic diurnal variation of serum cortisol. A dose schedule of 2 to 4 times daily may be appropriate for acute asthma but is usually not necessary for continuous corticosteroid therapy.

The asthma of some patients may be difficult to control even with high doses of continuous oral corticosteroids. These patients are thought to have "steroid-resistant asthma." These are very difficult cases that have few good therapeutic options.

Patients on continuous corticosteroid therapy should be managed for the development of clinically significant adverse effects. Periodic assessment may include monitoring of blood pressure, height, weight, glucose, electrolytes, and bone density, as well as evaluation for cataracts. Some patients may benefit from a preventive approach (such as vitamin D and supplemental calcium). Daily elemental calcium intake should be 1200 to 1500 mg; a suggested vitamin D daily dose is about 2500 IU.

Other Medications

Many other medications have been studied for their effects on asthma, particularly severe asthma. Such medications include methotrexate, cyclosporin, intravenous gamma-globulin, and inhaled lidocaine. None of these agents is approved for use in asthma, and their efficacy and safety in asthma have not been proven.

Key Points

Asthma medications can be divided into two major categories: quick-relief medications (medications used on an "as-needed" basis for symptom relief) and long-term control medications (medications for daily use to control inflammation and prevent airway remodeling).

- All patients with asthma should have a short-acting bronchodilator for as-needed use.

- Long-acting beta-agonists are used in combination with inhaled corticosteroids for patients with moderate or severe persistent asthma.

- Inhaled corticosteroids have broad anti-inflammatory effects and are highly effective in the treatment of chronic asthma. They are first-line therapy for all patients with persistent asthma.

- Patients with asthma that is not fully controlled by low- or medium-dose inhaled corticosteroids should use a combination of the inhaled corticosteroid with a long-acting beta-agonist, leukotriene modifier, or theophylline.

- Oral corticosteroids are used to treat acute asthma and severe persistent asthma that is not well controlled by inhaled corticosteroids and other agents.

▓   ▓   ▓

REFERENCES

1. **National Asthma Education and Prevention Program.** Expert Panel Report No. 2: Guidelines for the Diagnosis and Management of Asthma. National Institutes of Health Publication 98-4051. Bethesda, MD; 1998.

2. **Dennis SM, Sharp SJ, Vickers MR, et al.** Regular inhaled salbutamol and asthma control. The TRUST Randomised Trial. Lancet. 2000;355:1675–9.

3. **Davies B, Brooks G, Devoy M.** The efficacy and safety of salmeterol compared to theophylline: meta-analysis of nine controlled studies. Respir Med. 1998; 92:256–63.

4. **Pauwels RA, Lofdahl CG, Postma DS, et al.** Effect of inhaled formoterol and budesonide on exacerbations of asthma. Formoterol and Corticosteroids Establishing Therapy (FACET) International Study Group [see Comments] [erratum appears in N Engl J Med. 1998;338:139]. N Engl J Med. 1997;337:1405–11.

5. **Nelson HS, Busse WW, Kerwin E, et al.** Fluticasone propionate/salmeterol combination provides more effective asthma control than low-dose inhaled corticosteroid plus montelukast. J Allergy Clin Immunol. 2000;106:1088–95.

6. **Lipworth BJ.** Systemic adverse effects of inhaled corticosteroid therapy: a systematic review and meta-analysis. Arch Intern Med. 1999;159:941–55.

7. **Thomson NC.** Asthma therapy: theophylline. Can Respir J. 1998;5(suppl A):60A–63A.

8. **Busse WW, McGill KA, Horwitz RJ.** Leukotriene pathway inhibitors in asthma and chronic obstructive pulmonary disease. Clin Exp Allergy. 1999; 29(suppl 2):110–5.

7

■   ■   ■

Immunotherapy in the Management of Asthma

Harold S. Nelson, MD

llergen immunotherapy was first introduced in 1911. Controlled studies have proven the treatment to be effective in both children and adults in both allergic rhinitis and asthma. These studies have defined adequate doses in terms of the major allergen of the sensitizer and have demonstrated immunologic changes that provide a logical explanation for the clinical response. Studies have also demonstrated that immunotherapy may have some preventive effects against further sensitization in children and the progression, in children, from rhinitis to asthma. Finally, studies have now confirmed that continuing improvement is seen in many patients for years after termination of an adequate course of treatment.

The Role of Allergy in Asthma

Sensitivity to Allergens as a Risk Factor for the Presence of Asthma

A remarkably consistent association between sensitization to particular aeroallergens and risk of asthma has been reported from a number of countries (1). In unselected populations, children who become sensitive to indoor allergens (house dust mites, cat and dog dander, and, in the very damp climate of New Zealand, the indoor fungus *Aspergillus*) are at increased risk for developing asthma. Of the outdoor aeroallergens tested, sensitivity to the spores of the seasonal fungus *Alternaria* but not pollens conveys an increased risk for developing asthma. Instead of asthma, sensitivity to pollen increases the risk for rhinitis.

Most epidemiologic studies have been conducted in children. What is the risk for asthma in the sensitized adult? Studies conducted in Bergen,

Norway, in an unselected 18- to 73-year-old population compared sensitization as measured by the radioallergosorbent test (RAST) with objective evidence of pulmonary disease. By multivariate analysis, sensitization to house dust mites but not to other allergens was significantly associated with reduced FEV_1. Furthermore, there was a dose response between levels of IgE to house dust mites and impairment of lung function. Sensitivity to house dust mites and other indoor, but not outdoor, allergens was also associated with increased bronchial responsiveness to inhaled methacholine in the same population.

In Northern Sweden a random sample of 1859 subjects, aged 20 to 46 years, was investigated for risk factors for asthma. Positive skin tests for cats and dogs were found to be independently associated with asthma (relative risk, 3.6) and bronchial hyperresponsiveness (relative risk, 2.0). In this cold climate, where significant levels of mite allergen would not be encountered, sensitivity to house dust mites was not a risk for asthma.

Relation of Asthma Symptoms to Levels of Allergen Exposure

Increased levels of house dust mite in the home are a risk factor for developing asthma and for increased symptoms in house dust mite sensitized patients with asthma. Both relationships have been reported in adults as well as in children.

In randomly selected patients with asthma who were positive on skin testing to house dust mites, the levels of house dust mite allergen in the subjects beds significantly correlated with bronchial hyper-responsiveness and peak expiratory flow variability and negatively with FEV_1. In a group of newly diagnosed house dust mite sensitive adults with asthma, the levels of house dust mite allergen in their mattresses correlated with the amount of medication they had been employing to control their asthma.

One hundred twenty-nine consecutive patients with onset of asthma between ages 18 and 60 years were selected because they were positive to cat or dog on prick skin testing. The 39 patients with cats or dogs in their homes were compared with the 90 patients without cats or dogs. Those with pets in the home had greater symptoms, greater use of inhaled steroids, lower pulmonary function, and more evidence of airway inflammation. Despite this, they were less apt to attribute their symptoms to animals.

Sensitivity to outdoor seasonal fungal spores has been repeatedly implicated in severe asthma. In England, deaths in young adults occurred primarily in July or August. Deaths in people aged 45 to 64 years exhibited two peaks of excess mortality, one from November to March, and a separate peak in August. In those aged 65 to 74 years there was a winter excess lasting from November to April but no summer peak. Certain fungal spores but not pollens peak in August in England. The data suggest that, in England, exposure to fungal spores is an important factor in deaths due to asthma in those under 65 years of age. The most likely explanation for the winter peak in those over 45 is viral infections and diagnostic transfer from bronchitis to asthma.

In Chicago, deaths due to asthma were found to correlate with the outdoor mold spore counts but not with pollen counts. A group of adolescent and young adult patients evaluated at the Mayo Clinic later experienced respiratory arrest secondary to asthma. All episodes occurred in patients who had been sensitive on skin testing to *Alternaria* (an outdoor mold whose spores peak during the summer and early fall), and all the episodes occurred during the *Alternaria* spore season.

Effect of Reduction in Allergen Exposure on the Symptoms and Underlying Inflammation of Asthma

The effectiveness of avoidance or reduction of allergen exposure on the symptoms of asthma as well as on the underlying inflammation has been repeatedly demonstrated (Case 7-1) (see Chapter 5).

Evidence for the Effectiveness of Allergy Immunotherapy in Bronchial Asthma

Meta-analyses have demonstrated the effectiveness of allergen immunotherapy in both allergic rhinitis and asthma (2). Representative examples of the response in allergic rhinitis are the studies in grass pollen sensitive patients conducted by Varney and by Doltz. The Varney study is impressive because it was conducted in patients selected for their failure to respond to symptomatic treatment. The continuation of this study has provided remarkable insights into the immunologic changes produced by allergen immunotherapy (3) in addition to providing the best evidence in a controlled study of persistence of benefit following termination of treatment (4). The study by Doltz, unlike so many double-blind studies, continued for 3 years and demonstrated the progressive improvement that occurs over the course of treatment with maintenance doses of extract.

There have been many studies of the effectiveness of allergen immunotherapy in bronchial asthma; some have shown little or no benefit, but most have demonstrated clinical improvement. A meta-analysis of the 20 double-blind, placebo-controlled studies reported in the English language literature between 1966 and 1990 revealed that overall the odds for symptomatic improvement with immunotherapy were 2.7 (95% CI, 1.7 to 4.4). For immunotherapy with house dust mite extract, which constituted 45% of all studies, the odds for reduction in medication use were 4.2 (95% CI, 2.2 to 7.9). Benefit from immunotherapy in asthma is not difficult to demonstrate if the patients are appropriately selected and the dose employed is adequate. This was demonstrated in double-blind, placebo-controlled studies by Olsen in adult patients allergic to house dust mites; by

CASE 7-1   *Reducing allergen exposure in conjunction with immunotherapy when treating an asthma patient sensitive to allergens*

A 34-year-old woman, a resident of upper New York State, presents with a history of childhood asthma that became less severe beginning in high school but has been progressively increasing in severity over the past 5 years. She is currently awakening with chest tightness, shortness of breath, and wheezing 2 nights per month and using her albuterol rescue inhaler 4 or 5 times a week. She relates accompanying nasal stuffiness and postnasal drainage, with sneezing and rhinorrhea occurring April to June and August through September. A cat has been present in the home for the last 8 years and has full range of the house. Physical examination reveals bogginess of the nasal mucosa. The lungs are clear to auscultation.

The preferred next steps are to perform spirometry to assess the severity of the patient's asthma and perform allergy skin testing to assess sensitivity to her two perennial allergen exposures, cat and house dust mite.

The patient's FEV_1 is 90% of predicted, increasing to 98% of predicted following inhaled albuterol. Prick skin testing is strongly positive for the house dust mite (*D. pteronyssinus*), cat, oak, timothy grass, and short ragweed.

Discussion

The first step should be reducing exposure to the allergens to which this patient is sensitive and exposed. Encasing the mattress and pillows with allergen-impermeable covers and washing the bedding in 130°F water once weekly are cost-effective measures for reducing house dust mite exposure. The only certainly effective method for reducing cat exposure is to remove the cat from the home. At the very least, the cat should not be allowed in the patient's bedroom. Although recommended by some, washing a cat once weekly does not appear to be an effective means of reducing cat dander exposure. House dust mite allergens are carried on particles too large to remain airborne; therefore an air-cleaning device does not help patients with house dust mite sensitivity. The effects of a HEPA filter in removing cat dander from the air are quickly nullified by dispersion of cat dander from reservoirs in the carpet and upholstered furniture if the cat is allowed into that room. Allergy immunotherapy with cat and house dust mite extracts has been proven to be effective in patients with asthma who are sensitive to these allergens.

Varney, who studied immunotherapy in a cat allergic population, using exposure to a house occupied by cats to test the effectiveness; and by Walker (5), who examined the effect of grass pollen immunotherapy on both rhinitis and asthma. The patients in the Olsen study, who received active immunotherapy, experienced fewer symptoms, required less medication (including inhaled corticosteroids), and had improved pulmonary function compared with the placebo group. The Varney patients, who received active treatment, had a 75% reduction in symptoms on cat exposure compared with no change in the placebo group. In the Walker study, the reduction in the active group compared with the placebo group was as follows: rhinitis symptoms, 49% versus 15%; medication use, 80% versus 18%; and chest symptoms, 90% versus 11%. Bronchial responsiveness increased by three doubling dilutions of methacholine during the season in the placebo group and was unchanged in the grass-treated group (5).

Duration of Immunotherapy and Persistence of Improvement

Many patients have remained on specific immunotherapy for prolonged periods of time, sometimes several decades. The need for this prolonged treatment has recently undergone systematic scrutiny. Three studies have examined the rate of relapse in patients in whom immunotherapy was discontinued after a good response, in two cases following 3 or 4 years and in the other following 1 to 5 years of treatment. In 108 patients treated for 3 years with rye grass extract with improvement in symptoms, there was a 30% relapse rate in the first 3 years after stopping treatment, with few additional subjects relapsing over the next 2 years. Thirty-two adult patients who were successfully treated with grass immunotherapy for 3 to 4 years were randomized to continue treatment with grass extract or to receive placebo injections (4). After three additional years there was no difference in the symptoms during the grass pollen season in the group who had stopped immunotherapy compared with the group who continued. Injections of house dust mite extracts were stopped in 40 patients aged 7 to 45 years who had become asymptomatic after 1 to 5 years of treatment. Fifty-five percent relapsed during 3 years of follow-up. Relapse occurred in 62% who had received less than 3 years of treatment and in 48% of those whose treatment had extended beyond 3 years.

Immunologic Response to Allergen Immunotherapy

Clearly, for allergen immunotherapy not only to improve all aspects of asthma but to have a continuing effect following its discontinuation, it must have an effect on the underlying mechanisms of sensitization and inflammation.

For years the emphasis of the immunologic response to immunotherapy was on IgG-blocking antibody. Although easily demonstrated, the IgG response never convincingly related to clinical improvement. The effect of immunotherapy on specific IgE also failed to correlate with improvement. Even though specific IgE levels eventually fall, they are generally unchanged, or even increased, at a time when clinical improvement can be demonstrated.

Just as avoidance of relevant allergens can reduce airway inflammation, so too can specific allergen immunotherapy (6). Controlled studies have demonstrated decreased numbers of mucosal mast cells, decreased influx of eosinophils into the nasal and bronchial secretions during the relevant allergen exposure, and decreased immediate and late responses to allergen in the skin, nose, and lower airways.

Recently, attention has turned to the effect of allergen immunotherapy on the T lymphocytes. In allergic asthma, CD4+ T lymphocytes mount a predominantly Th_2-type response to inhalant allergens. This is characterized by the release of IL-4 and related cytokines rather than interferon-gamma, which is characteristic of the Th_1 phenotypic response. The cytokines released by the Th_2 lymphocytes promote infiltration and activation of eosinophils that are thought to be the primary effector cells in allergic inflammation. IL-4 also promotes a switch to production of allergen-specific IgE by B lymphocytes. The specific IgE sensitizes mast cells in the bronchial epithelium causing them, on contact with allergen, to release a variety of mediators and cytokines that contribute to the pathophysiology of asthma. Studies have demonstrated that allergen immunotherapy is associated with a shift from a Th_2 cytokine response, characterized by IL-4 production, to a Th_1 response, with predominance of interferon-gamma (3). For the first time, immunologic changes are being demonstrated that correlate with clinical improvement.

Practical Considerations in Immunotherapy

Selection of the Patient

The National Heart, Blood and Lung Institute's *Guidelines for the Diagnosis and Management of Asthma* state that allergen immunotherapy may be considered for asthma patients when

1. There is a clear evidence of a relationship between symptoms and exposure to an unavoidable allergen to which the patient is sensitive.
2. Symptoms occur all year or during a major portion of the year.
3. There is difficulty controlling symptoms with pharmacologic management because the medication is ineffective, multiple medications are required, or the patient is not accepting of medication.

There are requirements that must be met before considering placing a patient with allergic asthma on immunotherapy:

1. The patient must have significant exposure to the allergen(s) being considered for immunotherapy. This may be established by history, as in the case of animal dander, by information from previous aeroallergen or house dust sampling in the locality, or by analysis of the patient's house dust for allergens.
2. The patient must have demonstrated a significant level of sensitivity to the allergen(s). Usually this will be a positive prick skin test or a positive

in vitro test of equivalent sensitivity. Immunotherapy, based on positive intradermal tests following a negative prick skin test to inhalant allergens, should be pursued only when unusual circumstances justify treatment.

3. The pattern of symptoms must conform to the pattern of exposure. Outdoor aeroallergens in most localities will have a seasonal variation. Therefore immunotherapy solely with seasonal aeroallergen extracts for perennial asthma without seasonal variation or immunotherapy with perennial allergens for strictly seasonal symptoms is usually not warranted (Case 7-2).

The effectiveness of specific immunotherapy in the treatment of allergic rhinitis and allergic asthma is supported by the published studies. What are the situations in which specific immunotherapy is not indicated? This question has been addressed in guidelines developed by the Canadian Society of Allergy and Clinical Immunology. It concluded that specific immunotherapy was *inappropriate* in the following circumstances:

1. When, despite positive immediate skin tests, there was no indication of an IgE-mediated basis for the symptoms or disease
2. In cases of urticaria or atopic dermatitis
3. In cases of severe uncontrolled asthma
4. In children younger than 5 years of age
5. If previous properly administered immunotherapy was unsuccessful
6. If there is no improvement after 2 years of immunotherapy
7. For longer than 5 years.

CASE 7-2   *Patient with allergies who is not a candidate for immunotherapy*

A 44-year-old man from Ohio presents with a 5-year history of shortness of breath and wheezing. Symptoms are perennial without seasonal increase. He also has had typical symptoms of rhinorrhea and nasal discharge since a teenager. These symptoms are increased in April and May and in August and September. He has no pets. Physical examination reveals boggy nasal mucosa. The lungs are clear to auscultation. Spirometry yields an FEV_1 of 66% of predicted increasing to 72% of predicted after inhaling albuterol. Skin prick tests are strongly positive for oak, grass, and ragweed, with the remainder negative.

Discussion

Is immunotherapy a treatment option for this patient's asthma? The answer is No. He is not allergic to any perennial allergen, and his asthma does not become worse during the seasons when the pollens to which he is sensitive are in the air. Therefore immunotherapy would only benefit his hay fever symptoms. Clearly, immunotherapy does work for asthma (2,5), but only if the patient's symptoms can be attributed to a significant exposure to an allergen to which he is sensitive.

Although all these recommendations have not been subjected to rigorous testing, they would appear to be reasonable. Further notes of caution have been raised by Jean Bousquet, a French allergist with extensive experience in immunotherapy with house dust mite extracts in patients with asthma. In Bousquet's experience the response to house dust mite sensitive asthma is related to the age of the patient, patients less than 20 years of age being three times as apt to benefit as those over 51 years. The likelihood of response is also much less in patients who have fixed airflow obstruction, patients with an FEV_1 <60% of predicted being less than one-fourth as apt to respond to immunotherapy as those with an FEV_1 >90% of predicted.

Practical Considerations in the Administration of Allergen Extracts

An allergy extract treatment set (sometimes called an *allergy vaccine*) is typically provided as a maintenance concentration and as two to five ten-fold dilutions of the maintenance vial that are used for the initial build-up to maintenance. Injections begin with the most dilute and proceed to the maintenance concentrations (Table 7-1).

During the build-up phase, injections may be given weekly or more often, but doses should not be increased if the interval is greater than 2 weeks. If the interval since the last injection is 3 to 4 weeks, the previous dose should be repeated; if 5 to 7 weeks, reduce by one dose; if more than 7 weeks, consult the prescribing physician. Once the patient has achieved the maintenance dose (usually 0.5 cc of the maintenance vial), the intervals between injections can be gradually extended. Injections should be given several times at weekly intervals, then every 2 weeks, and finally every 4 weeks. Exceptions to the latter include patients allergic to pets in the home and patients during their first pollen season on maintenance. In these situations, more frequent injections sometimes appear to be more effective.

Table 7-1   Representative Schedule for Allergy Immunotherapy

1000-fold Dilution (cc)	100-fold Dilution (cc)	10-fold Dilution (cc)	Maintenance Concentration (cc)
0.05	0.05	0.05	0.05
0.10	0.10	0.07	0.07
0.20	0.20	0.10	0.10
0.40	0.40	0.15	0.15
		0.25	0.20
		0.35	0.30
		0.50	0.40
			0.50

Local reactions may be annoying and even painful. However, they do not appear to predict systemic reactions to subsequent injections. Therefore dosage modifications due to local reactions are made only for patient comfort. Premedication with a nonsedating antihistamine may reduce local and even systemic reactions.

Systemic reactions can range from mild rhinitis or asthma symptoms, to generalized itching and urticaria, to symptoms of abdominal cramping, hypotension, collapse, and death. For all except the mild respiratory reactions, epinephrine 1:1000 0.01 mL/kg to a maximum of 0.3 mL should be administered *intramuscularly* (to hasten absorption) and repeated at 5 to 10 min intervals as needed. Additional treatment may include inhaled short-acting bronchodilators and antihistamines. Oxygen and plasma expanders may be required for severe reactions.

Following a mild systemic reaction (mild asthma or rhinitis), return the patient to the previous dose. If this is tolerated, resume increases in dosage. For more severe reactions, the dosage is generally reduced by two doses below the one that caused the systemic reaction, then the doses are increased according to the schedule.

Because patients with asthma are more susceptible to systemic reactions than patients with rhinitis alone, and because the most common reaction asthma patients experience is bronchospasm, it is recommended that they be monitored with peak flow determinations before and after each injection. If their pre-injection peak flow is reduced, or if they are having symptoms that suggest their asthma is not under good control, they should not receive an injection. The peak flow should be repeated again before they leave the clinic after their injection (20 to 30 min). If the value has declined as much as 10%, they should be treated and further observed. Patients with significant fixed airflow obstruction are thought to be less likely to respond to allergen immunotherapy. Patients with poorly controlled asthma are particularly at risk for severe and even fatal bronchoconstriction as a reaction to their allergen injection. Also, patients with reduced lung function are more at risk, because they are less able to tolerate further bronchoconstriction. For all these reasons, it has become a common practice not to administer allergen immunotherapy to patients whose FEV_1 is less than 70% of predicted.

Another group of patients who are at particular risk for reactions to allergy immunotherapy are those receiving beta-adrenergic blocking agents. Not only are they more susceptible to reactions, but the reactions may be more difficult to treat. For this reason, use of beta-adrenergic blockers is usually considered a contraindication to receiving allergen immunotherapy.

Allergy Extracts

Allergy extracts, which are commercially available in the United States, are of three kinds: aqueous, 50% glycerin, and alum precipitated. They are prepared simply by adding the source of the allergen (field-collected pollen, animal hair and dander or pelt, or house dust mites or fungi grown in culture) to an extracting fluid. The mixture is allowed to sit for a time while the water-soluble proteins enter solution. The liquid is then removed and filtered for purity and sterilization. Glycerin may be added to enhance the stability of the proteins in solution but causes pain when injected. The proteins may be precipitated with aluminum hydroxide to provide a depot effect that decreases systemic reactions.

The resulting extract, if unstandardized, may be given one of two measures of potency. Weight-by-volume (w/v) indicates the weight of the initial allergenic material in grams divided by the volume of extracting fluid in milliliters. The alternative designation, protein nitrogen units (PNU), is based on the total protein contained in the final extract solution. The protein measured, however, is the total and not that which is allergenic (the latter may make up only a small percent of the total protein in solution). As might be expected, neither potency as weight-by-volume nor as protein nitrogen units bears a reliable relationship to allergenic potency of an extract. Unstandardized extracts with the same designation of potency will vary from manufacturer to manufacturer and even from lot to lot, depending on the allergen content of the raw material, as well as the conditions of extraction employed. The advantages of having standardized and hence consistent potency extracts are evident (Table 7-2).

Effective Dosing with Standardized Extracts

A number of double-blind, placebo-controlled studies have established effective doses for allergen immunotherapy. For the most part, these studies have been performed with extracts standardized by their content of their major allergen, rather than any of the methods of indicating potency used in the United States (see Table 7-2). However, data are available on the range of major allergen content found in a representative sample of commercial extracts produced in the United States (Table 7-3). This allows an approximation of the dosing that has proven to be effective in controlled studies.

Table 7-2 Advantages of Standardized Extracts

- Less manufacturer-to-manufacturer and lot-to-lot variation

- The ability to develop meaningful schedules for use of allergy extracts for diagnostic testing and immunotherapy

- The ability to compare skin test results from patient to patient and in the same patient over time

- Greater safety of immunotherapy in those patients who are appropriately treated with high-dose immunotherapy that is near the threshold for systemic reactions

Table 7-3   Effective Immunotherapy Dosing by Content of Major Allergy

Extract	Major Allergen	Effective Dose (μg)
Grass		
Timothy	Phl p 5	18
Ragweed		
Short ragweed	Amb a 1	12
House dust mites		
D. pteronyssinus	Der p 1	7
D. farinae	Der f 1	10
Cat	Fel d 1	15

Safety Considerations

Allergy immunotherapy, although offering an attractive treatment for many patients, has its limitations. Clearly, it is only effective to the extent that patient symptoms are produced by an IgE-mediated allergic reaction. Perhaps for this reason it is most predictably effective in younger patients. Not only is there more apt to be a significant nonallergic component in the older patients but also, in those with asthma, there may be a significant element of fixed airflow obstruction.

In addition to the cost and inconvenience of specific immunotherapy, there is the consideration of safety. Reactions vary from uncomfortable local swellings to systemic reactions that, rarely, may be fatal.

Local reactions may be troubling to the patient but do not seem to predict the occurrence of systemic reactions. Systemic reactions occur at differing rates, depending on patient and treatment variables. One review of 4810 patients receiving over 500,000 injections reported that 2.9% of the patients experienced a systemic reaction, none fatal. Systemic reactions in this report were most often related to grass pollen extracts and next most often to ragweed. Systemic reactions occurred most commonly in 10- to 39-year-olds, in women, and in highly sensitive patients. In those receiving injections of pollen extract, systemic reactions did not occur more commonly during that pollen season.

Seventeen fatal reactions to specific immunotherapy were reported in the United States during a 5-year period (1985-89). This represented approximately one fatality per 2.8 million injections. From the available data certain findings emerge: 87% of deaths occurred in patients who had asthma, and in all but one of these patients the asthma was severe or unstable. Most fatal reactions occurred during the build-up phase. Additional factors such as injection from a new bottle of extract, dosing errors, or administration when patients were symptomatic with asthma were frequently present.

Future of Allergen Immunotherapy

The risk as well as the inconvenience of injection immunotherapy has led some investigators, particularly in Europe, to try intranasal and sublingual-oral immunotherapy. Both of these approaches are safe and effective if adequate doses are employed. The sublingual-oral therapy employed in Europe must be differentiated from the homeopathic dosing by this route often employed in the United States.

Allergen immunotherapy, although effective, has been to a degree displaced by symptomatic therapy for bronchial asthma and allergic rhinitis. A major reason for its loss of popularity is the prolonged course of the treatment and the occurrence of reactions, both of which are due to the reaction of the allergenic extract with IgE. Thanks to recombinant technology, the possibility exists of modifying the major allergens so that they have reduced reactivity with IgE. Furthermore, the recombinant allergens can be combined with immunostimulatory DNA sequences that favor the transformation from the Th_2 phenotype characteristic of allergy to a Th_1 cytokine profile. Thus recombinant technology and new understanding of ways to alter the immune response to allergens promise to make allergy immunotherapy safer and more effective.

Conclusion

For allergen immunotherapy to be effective

1. The allergy must make a significant contribution to the asthmatic patient's symptoms.
2. The relevant allergens must be administered in adequate doses.
3. High-dose immunotherapy must be administered for an appropriate period of time (generally 3 to 5 years).

If these conditions are met, allergen immunotherapy is an effective treatment for allergic rhinitis and asthma that, uniquely, offers the possibility of persisting improvement after treatment is stopped. Therefore allergen immunotherapy should be considered as a possible adjunct to symptomatic treatment in asthmatic patients with allergic respiratory diseases. Its use should not be limited to those asthmatic patients failing symptomatic therapy.

■   ■   ■

Key Points

- Sensitivity to indoor allergens (e.g., house dust mites) rather than outdoor allergens is a risk factor for asthma.

- The recommended duration of immunotherapy is 3 to 5 years. Symptoms remain improved in most patients after immunotherapy of this duration is discontinued.

- Immunotherapy may be considered for patients with asthma only if the patient's symptoms are largely caused by an unavoidable allergen, the symptoms occur at least during most of the year, and the patient has been unable to easily control symptoms with pharmacologic therapy.

- Local reactions to the allergen extract may occur, but these are not predictive of systemic reactions.

- Asthmatic patients should be monitored with peak flow determinations before and after each injection to avoid bronchospasm as a reaction to the treatment. Patients with poorly controlled asthma and reduced lung function are particularly at risk for severe or fatal bronchoconstriction.

■   ■   ■

REFERENCES

1. **Nelson HS.** Does allergen immunotherapy have a role in the treatment of bronchial asthma? Allergy Asthma Proc. 1997;18:157–62.

2. **Abramson MJ, Puy RM, Weiner JM.** Is allergen immunotherapy effective in asthma? A meta-analysis of randomized controlled trials. Am J Respir Crit Care Med. 1995;151:969–74.

3. **Durham SR, Till SJ.** Immunologic changes associated with allergen immunotherapy. J Allergy Clin Immunol. 1998;102:157–64.

4. **Durham SR, Walker SM, Varga E-M, et al.** Long-term clinical efficacy of grass-pollen immunotherapy. N Engl J Med. 1999;341:468–75.

5. **Walker SM, Pajno GB, Lima MT, et al.** Grass pollen immunotherapy for seasonal rhinitis and asthma: a randomized, controlled trial. J Allergy Clin Immunol. 2001;107:87–93.

6. **Nelson HS.** Immunotherapy for inhalant allergens. In: Middleton E Jr, Reed CE, Ellis EF, et al, eds. Allergy: Principles and Practice, 5th ed. St. Louis: Mosby-Year Book; 1998:1050–62.

8

■ ■ ■

Exercise-Induced Asthma

Mark T. O'Hollaren, MD

E xercise-induced asthma (EIA), also known as exercise-induced bronchospasm, is a term used to describe asthmatic symptoms of cough, shortness of breath, wheezing, and/or chest tightness experienced in association with physical exertion. Exercise-induced asthma occurs with equal frequency in both children and adults, and if unrecognized and untreated, may significantly restrict an individual's ability to exercise (1,2). This transient increase in airways resistance during or following exercise occurs in 80% to 90% of patients with asthma; however, nearly all patients with asthma will experience symptoms of EIA with an exercise challenge of significant magnitude (1,3). Approximately 40% of patients with allergic rhinitis will also experience EIA, and the prevalence in the general population is between 6% and 13% (3). Nine percent of patients with EIA have no history of asthma or allergic disease (3).

Exercise-induced asthma is frequently unrecognized, even among elite (e.g., Olympic level) athletes. The incidence may vary significantly among athletes of different sporting events. For example, in studies of the United States Olympic teams, the incidence of EIA in cross-country skiers, mountain bikers, and cyclists has been reported to be as high as 50%, whereas almost no EIA was found among competitive divers and weight lifters (4,5). In a study of Olympic athletes competing in the 1996 summer games, the incidence of EIA across all sports was 16.6%, which was higher than that of the 1984 summer games (5). A similar study of athletes competing in the winter Olympics found a 23% overall incidence of EIA across all sports and genders, with the highest incidence in cross-country skiers (4). These differences suggest that the presence of EIA may influence the sport in which an athlete chooses to compete.

Cultural and social factors may also influence EIA. Studies of high school football players have shown a higher incidence of EIA among athletes of

African-American descent compared with those of European descent, as well as a higher incidence in those who live in poverty.

Patients experiencing exercise-induced asthma may complain of chest tightness, shortness of breath, cough, and/or audible wheezing either with exercise or within a few minutes after exercise (Table 8-1). These symptoms are the same as those experienced by patients with asthma, although the symptoms of EIA are usually of shorter duration. Dyspnea due to undiagnosed EIA is frequently falsely attributed to being "out of shape" (Case 8-1).

Table 8-1   Clinical Characteristics of Exercise-Induced Asthma

Symptoms
  Cough
  Shortness of breath
  Chest tightness
  Audible wheezing

Timing of Symptoms
  Symptoms usually begin during exercise, limiting its duration and/or intensity,
    and usually peak in the 5 to 15 min following its completion

---

CASE 8-1   *Patient with exercise-induced asthma: the "out-of-shape" label*

A 15-year-old high school sophomore is brought in by his father because he is not keeping up with the rest of the junior varsity basketball team. The coach has suggested a visit to the doctor, although the father is convinced that he simply needs to buckle down and get into better shape.

The patient has no chest complaints at times other than when he exercises, and then he reports that it feels as if he "can't get enough air." About 10 min into basketball practice he notes some coughing, chest tightness, and shortness of breath. If he continues to run up and down the court, he hears wheezing. He says that he is not able to keep up with his teammates during practices and games.

The patient saw his general internist, who noted normal cardiovascular and lung examinations. Spirometry showed an FEV_1 of 98% predicted and an FVC of 100% predicted. His PEFR was normal at 500 L/min. He was given a peak flow meter to use before exercise, with instructions to recheck his PEFR when he became symptomatic and 5 min after completing exercise. His physician also gave him an albuterol inhaler to use if needed.

The patient noted that his PEFR fell from 500 L/min pre-exercise to 390 L/min during exercise and to 370 L/min measured 5 min after completion of exercise. The following day, he took inhaled albuterol 2 puffs immediately before practice and was able to exercise without problems. PEFR was 480 L/min before exercise and did not change with exercise. He has since been able to exercise without problems with pretreatment with inhaled albuterol.

Most commonly, symptoms of EIA are short-lived and remit with either treatment or cessation of exercise. On occasion, however, EIA may be severe, and fatalities have occurred. It is not possible to predict how much pulmonary function will fall with exercise based on the value of a resting FEV_1. Patients who have normal resting lung function can have severe falls in pulmonary function with exercise (1).

Appropriate recognition and treatment of EIA is important for several reasons. First, a timely diagnosis allows for appropriate relief of the patient's respiratory symptoms. Secondly, proper treatment may eliminate the negative effects of the patient's desire to avoid the symptoms of EIA by refraining completely from all physical exercise. Those patients who eliminate or reduce their exercise routines due to breathing difficulties will lose out on the salutary effects of regular exercise. Exercise is important for the maintenance of general health, weight reduction, stress relief, cardiac rehabilitation, and control of other medical conditions such as hypertension and diabetes. Furthermore, children and adolescents with impaired exercise tolerance may not be able to participate fully in sports or recreational activities with their peers, and may thus feel they are "different" or that they "don't measure up" to others in their age group. This may in turn make younger patients with asthma lose self-esteem and discourage them from participating in sports. They may also lose out on the social and psychological benefits accrued from participating as a member of a team.

It is not uncommon for EIA to go undiagnosed for years. Patients experiencing dyspnea with exertion may delay seeking medical help, assuming that their respiratory symptoms are due to poor physical fitness, which is unfortunate because this disorder is readily treatable.

In contrast to many other medical problems of childhood, someone outside of the immediate family may first suggest the possibility of EIA. It is very common for younger patients with EIA to have the diagnosis pointed out by a coach or physical education teacher, who may observe that a particular individual consistently coughs with exercise or lags behind the rest of a group in exercises such as running for prolonged distances. For these reasons, an awareness of the typical and less typical presentations of EIA is important for physicians who treat younger patients and adults with respiratory complaints.

Pathophysiology and Etiology

An understanding of the pathophysiology of EIA is helpful to most effectively recognize and treat this disorder. The airway narrowing, which occurs following moderate to severe episodes of EIA, leads to a mismatch in pulmonary ventilation and perfusion, with a subsequent decrease in arterial oxygen tension (1).

During the first few minutes of exercise, bronchodilation occurs in most individuals, whether or not they have asthma. This transient improvement in airway caliber may be more dramatic in patients with moderate or severe airway obstruction (e.g., asthma and cystic fibrosis) (1). As exercise continues in patients with EIA, this bronchodilation may give way to bronchoconstriction. This bronchoconstriction may occur during exercise, (especially prolonged exercise), but tends to be most severe in the 5 to 15 min following completion of exercise. The reasons for this delayed onset are unclear. Some argue that the hyperpnea accompanying increased minute ventilation may protect the airways during exercise, whereas others believe that the airway cooling seen with exercise may be protective and the rewarming that accompanies cessation of exercise may trigger bronchospasm (6). The airway water and heat loss hypothesized to trigger EIA is discussed in more detail below. Some investigators believe that EIA is multifactorial in origin, and that bronchial blood flow, which may be increased in patients with asthma, may be responsible for the altered thermoregulation leading to EIA (1).

In addition to EIA symptoms occurring during or immediately following exercise, some patients with EIA will also experience a delayed asthmatic response, occurring several hours after exercise. In children, this late bronchospastic response occurs more commonly in those who have experienced a late asthmatic response to allergen challenge. There are insufficient data available to assess this association between late asthmatic response to allergen and its relationship to late exercise-associated asthmatic responses in adults. This association in children is in keeping with the observation that patients who experience a delayed asthmatic response to inhaled allergen frequently have residual increased bronchial hyper-responsiveness to nonspecific stimuli such as exercise. The late asthmatic response to exercise itself, however, does not appear to consistently increase bronchial hyper-responsiveness, as measured by the response to inhaled histamine, methacholine, or isocapnic hyperventilation.

The amount of respiratory ventilation, as well as the humidity and temperature of the inspired air, are important factors in determining the severity of exercise-induced asthma. It has long been known that exercising in cold dry air (such as with cross-country skiing) results in more severe EIA symptoms than when exercising in warm moist air (such as with indoor swimming). These findings have led to a number of observations and theories concerning the role of respiratory water and heat loss and the causation of EIA.

Under normal resting breathing conditions, the majority of the warming and humidification of inspired air is done by the nasal mucosa. However, during vigorous exercise, the large airways are recruited to provide the extra heat and humidity to condition the inspired air (1). Carbon dioxide and water vapor are among the expiratory products of the respiratory cycle. As an individual exercises, minute ventilation and, therefore, respiratory water and heat loss increase. The amount of expired water vapor lost from the moist lining of the bronchial tree and lung tissue may be affected by the ambient humidity of the inspired air. Inhalation of moist warm air results in less exhaled respiratory water and heat loss than does inspiring cold dry air.

In addition to evaporative water loss during exercise, airway cooling also takes place. Energy is required for water to be converted from a liquid (lining the airway walls) to exhaled water vapor. More than 80% of the energy required for this conversion of water from the airway surfaces into water vapor is obtained in the form of heat taken from the airway wall. This evaporative cooling of the airway was originally thought to be the primary cause of EIA, because experimental data showed that EIA was often inhibited or prevented by inspiring fully saturated air at body temperature and increased with inspiration of cold dry air (1,7). There is still some disagreement among experts in the field regarding the relative contributions of airway water loss versus airway cooling (or both) in the causation of EIA. It is difficult to separate the role of these two potential triggers of EIA, but many investigators currently believe that water loss is the principal trigger of EIA. In support of this theory, experimental inhalation of hot dry air (which results in significantly less airway cooling) still can produce EIA, although there may still be some cooling through evaporative heat loss in this setting (1).

Others have looked at potential alternative explanations for EIA, including an increase in gastroesophageal reflux accompanying exercise or an increase in acute airway inflammation as measured by exhaled nitric oxide; however, no significant evidence supports these mechanisms as explanations for EIA.

Another interesting observation is that approximately 50% of patients who have EIA will be refractory (or partially refractory) to EIA if they exercise again within 60 min of the first exercise session (1). There may still, however, be a smaller but significant fall in FEV_1 with the second exercise challenge. If the second exercise challenge is more than 3 hr after the first, the refractory period is lost, and the fall in pulmonary function (peak expiratory flow rate or FEV_1) will be similar to that seen after the first exercise challenge (1). This refractory period does not occur if the patient is pretreated with indomethacin, arguing that prostaglandins (such as prostaglandin E-2) may be playing a role in airway protection during the refractory period following exercise (1).

Finally, urinary excretion of the leukotriene LTE-4 increases after exercise, although the amount excreted does not appear to correlate with the degree of bronchospasm. This excretion of urinary leukotrienes is significantly decreased with pretreatment with montelukast, a potent cysteinyl leukotriene receptor antagonist that is effective in preventing EIA.

Diagnosis

In some cases of EIA the diagnosis may be fairly clear from the clinical history, whereas in others diagnosis may be more difficult to establish. It is clear that in many patients the diagnosis may be missed for years. The usual symptoms experienced by patients with EIA may be any or all of the following: cough, shortness of breath, chest tightness, and audible wheezing. As mentioned earlier, symptoms may occur during exercise or within the first 5 to 15 min after completion of exercise. They typically clear within 60 min after completion of exercise, and the patient may state that he or she is able to exercise for 1 to 2 hr afterwards with few or no symptoms of EIA. If the patient waits more than 3 hr after an episode of EIA, however, the symptoms return in their usual fashion.

Symptoms are usually more pronounced with aerobic exercise, which involves a significant increase in the ventilatory rate (e.g., running or cross-country skiing) compared with those that do not require as high a ventilatory rate (e.g., weight lifting or competitive diving). Patients usually state that symptoms are especially notable when exercising in cold dry air compared with warmer moist air. It should be noted, however, that self-reported symptoms of EIA have not been shown to be completely reliable, at least in elite athletes.

Exercise-induced hyperventilation with hypocapnea may produce symptoms similar to EIA. These patients (frequently children and adolescents) may experience chest discomfort and be misdiagnosed as EIA but have very little, if any, fall in FEV_1 (8). Post-exercise cough is also a common symptom of EIA, but cough with exercise may occur separate and distinct from EIA. Exercise-induced cough has a time course similar to EIA, but is not accompanied by a fall in PEFR or FEV_1. Exercise-induced cough may not respond to standard doses of albuterol or cromolyn. Occasionally, an athlete may present with symptoms that are consistent with a diagnosis of EIA but does not respond to treatment. Further investigation of such patients may lead to a totally different diagnosis (e.g., vocal cord dysfunction).

In the laboratory, EIA is diagnosed with a 10% fall in PEFR or FEV_1, or a 35% fall in FEF_{25-75} or specific conductance (S_{gaw}) (1). In the physician's office, a 15% or greater fall from the pre-exercise value is typically used (3). When evaluating a patient for possible EIA, objective measures of airway function with exercise are very helpful in establishing the diagnosis. An exercise trial on either a treadmill or a stationary bicycle has been used. Clinicians have also had patients run up and down the stairs of their office building or run outdoors for a period of time. A tactic of some referral centers has been to have a separate supply of chilled dry air for use during the indoor exercise challenge. Because of the airway heat and water loss using this technique, this maximizes the chance of an asthmatic response with exercise.

A pre-exercise value of either PEFR or FEV_1 should be at least 75% of either the patient's predicted value or 75% of personal best. Measurements should be taken immediately after completion of exercise and at 1, 3, 5, and 10 min after stopping exercise. The lowest post-exercise value (usually obtained between 3 and 12 min after completion of exercise) is then obtained. The percent fall is calculated by subtracting the lowest pulmonary function value from the pre-exercise value and expressing it as a percent of the pre-exercise value (1). Although most patients experience their most noticeable symptoms in the 10 min or so after exercise has stopped, some individuals experience their most severe symptoms during exercise (9).

In cases where the diagnosis is still unclear despite attempts to measure pulmonary function, and patients are not responding to therapy, further evaluation is needed. Medical evaluation may be indicated to ensure that no other pulmonary or cardiac pathology exists. Formal exercise testing in a referral facility may also be useful in establishing the diagnosis. This may involve spirometry with lung volumes, diffusion capacity, and oxygen saturation with exercise, as well as laryngoscopy when symptoms are present (to rule out exercise-induced vocal cord dysfunction).

Finally, investigation into possible allergic triggers of the patient's underlying asthma may be very revealing, and appropriate skin testing, allergen avoidance measures, and allergen immunotherapy may be very useful for overall asthma control in some patients (Case 8-2).

A suggested approach to the diagnosis of EIA is given in Table 8-2.

CASE 8-2   *Patient with exercise-induced asthma: the allergy factor*

Melissa is a 23-year-old marathon runner who, despite her long history of rigorous training, has been disappointed with her running times, stating that she "can't get to the next level of fitness" because of waxing and waning shortness of breath. She has made several observations. First, she notes that her breathing tends to be better if she does prolonged mild exercise (i.e., a very light jog) for 5 to 10 min before she does her regular run. Second, she has noted that her breathing is clearly worse when the weather is cold outside or if she runs in more arid locations, especially during the winter.

Her doctor previously suspected EIA and gave her an albuterol inhaler for use before exercise. Although the inhaler seemed to help somewhat, her symptoms continued, especially after about mile 5 when she is running a prolonged distance.

Her history was also notable for a pet cat, which slept on her bed at night; a feather pillow and comforter were also on her bed. Spirometry showed an FEV_1 of 72% predicted and an FVC of 86% predicted, with a 9% improvement after inhaled bronchodilators.

Melissa was referred for allergy consultation and was found to be allergic to cat and dust mite. Appropriate allergen avoidance measures were initiated, with her cat moved outside, allergen-proof encasings placed over her bed, etc. She was put on inhaled corticosteroids and salmeterol. Her exercise tolerance improved significantly but still fell somewhat short of what she considered her potential, and PEFR confirmed a continued 15% fall with exertion. After montelukast was added to her regimen she had complete clearance of her EIA symptoms and was able to vigorously pursue competitive running.

Table 8-2   Suggested Approach to the Diagnosis of Exercise-Induced Asthma

---

1. Take a careful clinical history to establish the relationship of symptoms with physical exertion. In patients with known asthma, the clinical picture of EIA is likely to be increased symptoms similar to their asthma symptoms at other times.

2. Provide the patient with a peak flow meter and obtain baseline measurements before exercise, immediately after completion of exercise, and at 1, 3, 5, and 10 min after stopping exercise. This is helpful in establishing the diagnosis when it is unclear. In patients with known asthma, measurement of peak expiratory flow rates (PEFRs) are useful for following response to treatment.

3. If the patient experiences symptoms of cough, chest tightness, shortness of breath, and/or audible wheezing, and PEFR falls by 15% or more following exercise, then a presumptive diagnosis of EIA may be made.

4. Assuming other medical causes of dyspnea on exertion are not suspected (or if suspected previously they have been ruled out), then a trial of EIA prophylaxis may be tried as outlined in Table 8-3.

Treatment

Nonpharmacologic Measures

There are a number of therapeutic modalities currently available to effectively treat exercise-induced asthma. First, whenever possible, patients should be advised to have a warm-up period before more strenuous exercise. During this time they may stretch, as well as perform some mild exercise for 5 to10 min. This easing into exercise may help decrease the severity of EIA in many athletes. Physical endurance training itself appears to have little or no effect on the severity of exercise-induced asthma (1). Because breathing warmed and humidified air is helpful in patients with EIA, nasal breathing has been advocated in these patients. This may be difficult, however, due to the large volume of air required during strenuous exercise and because many of these patients also have nasal disease (1).

Pharmacologic Measures

The mainstay of treatment for EIA is pharmacotherapy. Inhaled beta-2 agonists are among the most effective drugs for preventing EIA and will reduce or eliminate EIA in approximately 90% of patients (1). Short-acting beta-agonists are the first-line choice for prophylaxis of EIA. Aerosol forms of beta-agonists have been shown to be clearly superior to oral formulations of these drugs (1). Two puffs of an inhaled short-acting beta-agonist (e.g., albuterol) will protect against EIA for approximately 2 hr, even though its duration of bronchodilation may last nearly 4 hr (1). Formulations of albuterol using an HFA propellant system have been shown to work equally as well as those using chlorofluorocarbon propellant systems in preventing EIA. Long-acting beta-agonists, such as salmeterol (Serevent) (2 inhalations), have also been shown to be effective in preventing EIA. They have the advantage of being able to be taken hours before exercise and maintaining their protective effect against EIA; however, the duration of action of salmeterol in preventing EIA may decrease slightly over time (10).

Inhaled cromolyn or nedocromil may be considered for patients in whom short-acting beta-agonists are not fully effective. Cromolyn or nedocromil is effective in approximately 80% of patients and nearly devoid of side effects; if ineffective, a somewhat higher dose may be tried. Both cromolyn and nedocromil are equally effective in adults and children; unlike albuterol, both will help prevent the late asthmatic response to exercise (1). Cromolyn or nedocromil, when used in combination with an inhaled beta-agonist, may have a synergistic effect. These inhalers work best when 2 inhalations are administered approximately 20 min before exercise but will also have some effectiveness even if taken immediately before.

The leukotriene antagonists are a new therapeutic class of medication effective for the prevention of EIA. Drugs such as montelukast (Singulair) and zafirlukast (Accolate) have been shown to effectively diminish or prevent EIA (10). In an 8-week double-blind randomized study comparing montelukast and salmeterol for prevention of EIA, both treatments were effective, although montelukast maintained protection over the full 8 weeks whereas salmeterol had some development of tolerance over that time (10).

An anticholinergic agent such as inhaled ipratropium bromide (2 puffs) may provide a slight benefit when taken before exercise. This drug appears to work, however, by causing some pre-exercise bronchodilation and does not appear to be as effective as other agents in this setting. It may be considered as add-on therapy for patients with severe EIA who are not responding to more traditionally used agents.

Inhaled corticosteroids have essentially no effect on EIA when taken before exercise, but may decrease the intensity of EIA if taken over several weeks, presumably by improving overall asthma control (1).

Drugs that inhibit the cyclooxygenase pathway (e.g., aspirin, nonsteroidal anti-inflammatory drugs) have no protective effect on EIA. However, indomethacin has been shown experimentally to block the late asthmatic response to exercise (1).

Although terfenadine (Seldane), which has been withdrawn from the US market, given in doses several times the usual therapeutic dose had some protective effect against EIA, no data support antihistamine use for the prevention or treatment of EIA.

Several other drugs have been used with varying levels of success for the treatment of EIA. Calcium-channel blockers have had some success in preventing EIA, and they may be considered as add-on therapy in patients who have failed beta-agonists in combination with cromolyn and/or

---

Table 8-3   Suggested Treatment Approach to Exercise-Induced Asthma

It is assumed with all treatment approaches that a period of stretching and warm-up exercises are undertaken for 5 to 10 min before commencing strenuous exercise.

1. Two puffs of albuterol taken from 0 to 20 min before exercise is effective in dramatically reducing or eliminating EIA in 80% to 90% of patients. If the inhaled form of albuterol (or another short-acting beta-agonist) is taken in a pressurized metered dose inhaler, the puffs should be taken one at a time, inhaled slowly to maximal inhalational capacity, and the breath held for 10 seconds with each puff.

2. If the patient continues to experience EIA symptoms despite pretreatment with albuterol, add two puffs of inhaled cromolyn or nedocromil to the inhaled albuterol 0 to 20 min before exercise.

3. If the patient does not achieve effective relief despite the above measures, several alternative approaches can be employed. If the patient has chronic asthma, it is essential that overall asthma control is achieved using accepted treatment guidelines (see Suggested Reading section at end of chapter). If inhaled short-acting beta-agonists and cromolyn or nedocromil are not effective, a trial of an inhaled long-acting beta-agonist or leukotriene modifier is indicated.

4. Evaluation of possible allergic triggers with appropriate skin testing, allergen avoidance education, and so on is indicated if symptoms persist.

---

leukotriene antagonists such as montelukast. Inhaled furosemide has been shown experimentally to be useful in preventing EIA, although it is not commercially available. A number of other drugs normally used for other purposes have been shown to occasionally be helpful, but do not appear to be clinically useful.

When assessing the success of a medical program for treating EIA, the physician may use a combination of subjective measures (e.g., how the patient's symptoms respond to exercise) and objective measures (e.g., measures of pulmonary function). Portable mechanical devices, such as a peak expiratory flow meter (PEFM), or electronic portable pulmonary function devices, such as the Airwatch portable pulmonary function device, are ideal for this purpose. Symptoms and peak expiratory flow rate measurements can be logged by the patient, and the response to various treatment regimens can be evaluated.

A suggested approach to treatment of EIA is given in Table 8-3.

Summary

Exercise-induced asthma is characterized by symptoms of cough, shortness of breath, chest tightness, and/or audible wheezing as a result of bronchoconstriction following physical exertion. The vast majority of patients with asthma experience increased asthma symptoms in response to exercise.

Exercise-induced asthma is most likely caused by a combination of evaporative water and heat loss from the airway wall, and may be minimized or eliminated by proper warm-up before exercise, combined with appropriate pharmacotherapy. Inhaled beta-agonists, cromolyn sodium, nedocromil, and leukotriene antagonists are all effective medications for preventing symptoms. The diagnosis of EIA is frequently missed, and a proper index of suspicion is needed by the treating physician because effective treatment is available that will allow these patients to substantially improve their quality of life.

Key Points

- Exercise-induced asthma is often undiagnosed for years because persons with the condition tend to attribute their symptoms to being "out of shape."

- Exercise-induced asthma is characterized by symptoms of cough, shortness of breath, chest tightness, and/or wheezing, occurring either during exercise or within the first 5 to 15 min after completion of exercise.

- The main factors in the causation of EIA are respiratory water and heat loss and evaporative cooling of the airway (which may be affected by the humidity and temperature of inspired air). Therefore EIA is more likely to occur in cold dry air.

- In patients with an appropriate history and symptoms, EIA is diagnosed with a 15% decrease in FEV_1 from the pre-exercise value.

- Pharmacotherapy is a mainstay of treatment of EIA, with short-acting inhaled beta-agonists being first-line agents. Proper "warm-ups" of mild exercise should be performed before more vigorous exercise.

REFERENCES

1. **Anderson SD.** Exercise-induced asthma. In: Middleton E, Reed CE, Ellis EF, et al, eds. Allergy: Principles and Practice, 4th ed. Philadelphia: Mosby-Year Book; 1993.
2. **Burr ML, Butland BK, King S, et al.** Changes in asthma prevalence: two surveys 15 years apart. Arch Dis Child. 1989;64:1452–6.
3. **Milgrom H, Taussig LM.** Keeping children with exercise-induced asthma active. Pediatrics. 1999;104:38.
4. **Wilber RL, Rundell KW, Szmedra L, et al.** Incidence of exercise-induced bronchospasm in Olympic winter sport athletes. Med Sci Sports Exerc. 2000;32:732–7.
5. **Weiler JM, Layton T, Hunt M.** Asthma in United States: Olympic athletes who participated in the 1996 summer games. J Allergy Clin Immunol. 1998;102:722–6.

6. **McFadden ER, Lenner KA, Strohl KP.** Postexertional airway rewarming and thermally induced asthma. J Clin Invest. 1986; 78:18–25.

7. **Chen WY, Horton DJ.** Heat and water loss from the airways and exercise-induced asthma. Respiration. 1977;34:305–13.

8. **Hammo AH, Weinberger MM.** Exercise-induced hyperventilation: a pseudo-asthma syndrome. Ann Allergy Asthma Immunol. 1999;82:574–8.

9. **Storms WW.** Exercise-induced asthma: diagnosis and treatment for the recreational or elite athlete. Med Sci Sports Exerc. 1999;31:S33–8.

10. **Edelman JM, Turpin JA, Bronsky EA, et al.** Oral montelukast compared with inhaled salmeterol to prevent exercise-induced bronchoconstriction: a randomized, double-blind trial. Exercise Study Group. Ann Intern Med. 2000;132: 97–104.

SUGGESTED READING

Allergy Report. American Academy of Allergy, Asthma, and Immunology; 2000. This document is also available at www.theallergyreport.org. (A consensus document of 21 national specialty, primary care, and lay organizations involved in the treatment of allergic diseases, the Allergy Report is a tremendous resource.)

Guidelines for the Diagnosis and Management of Asthma. Bethesda, MD: National Institutes of Health. NIH Publication 97-4051; 1997.

9

■ ■ ■

Interrelationships Between the
Upper and Lower Airways

Raymond G. Slavin, MD

t is often the assumption that the upper and lower airways are anatomically and physiologically separate and distinct entities. There are, however, important relationships between the two. Specifically, diseases of the upper airways can impact unfavorably on the lower airways and worsen asthma. Treatment of upper airway disease will also frequently result in improvement in asthma. This chapter deals with two upper airway diseases, rhinitis and sinusitis, and their relationships to asthma.

Rhinitis

Allergic rhinitis is an extremely common disease, affecting more than 40 million Americans. It has proven to be quite costly, both directly in terms of dollars spent and indirectly in terms of life-style impact. Allergic rhinitis is characteristically associated with several comorbidities including allergic conjunctivitis, sinusitis, otitis media, and asthma.

Association of Rhinitis and Asthma

There are a number of studies clearly showing the significant association of allergic rhinitis and asthma (Table 9-1). Up to 58% of patients with rhinitis have diagnosed asthma. In one database analysis of asthma, the prevalence of rhinitis ranged between 85% and 95%. There is also evidence that patients with asthma who deny symptoms of rhinitis have inflammatory changes in their nasal mucosa. Therefore, one may argue that, in most patients with asthma, the entire respiratory tract is involved. This has prompted

---

Table 9-1   Interrelationships Between Allergic Rhinitis and Asthma

---

- Allergic rhinitis and asthma frequently co-exist
- Allergic rhinitis is a risk factor for developing asthma
- Rhinitis makes asthma worse
- Asthma makes rhinitis worse
- Nasal dysfunction causes changes in lower airway function

---

the introduction of the term *chronic allergic airways syndrome* (1). At the lower end of the spectrum are patients with upper airway disease alone, whereas the high end consists of patients with both rhinitis and asthma.

Nonallergic rhinitis has also been found to be associated with asthma (2). In a recent study, patients with perennial rhinitis had almost four times the incidence of asthma as patients with no rhinitis.

Another example of co-morbidity of rhinitis and asthma occurs in patients sensitive to aspirin and nonsteroidal anti-inflammatory drugs. In the workplace, symptoms of rhinitis are commonly associated with occupational asthma. For example, one study showed 92% of subjects with occupational asthma experienced rhinitis symptoms.

Given these examples, it can be stated that both allergic and nonallergic rhinitis are strongly associated with asthma.

Rhinitis as a Risk Factor for Asthma

A group of Brown University freshmen were skin tested and evaluated for allergy. None of them had asthma. Some of the group had allergic rhinitis and were skin test positive; the rest were negative by history and skin testing. A 23-year follow-up questionnaire revealed that the group who had allergic rhinitis as freshmen had developed asthma three times more frequently than those with no history of allergic rhinitis. Of the group who developed asthma, 86% also had allergic rhinitis. Among the participants with both asthma and seasonal allergic rhinitis, 44.8% experienced the development of seasonal allergic rhinitis first, 34.5% experienced the development of asthma first, and 20.7% experienced the development of both diseases at the same time (3). In addition to this study, a 15-year study on adult twins in Finland showed that seasonal allergic rhinitis was usually diagnosed before asthma and considerably increased the risk of asthma.

Impact of Rhinitis on Asthma Severity

There appears to be evidence of increased symptom severity, involving the entire respiratory tract, in patients with both rhinitis and asthma. In patients with more severe rhinitis, a number of asthma parameters are worsened, including weekly attacks, nocturnal awakenings, and work loss. Rhinitis

---

Table 9-2   Similarities Between the Upper and Lower Airways

- Anatomic
  Continuous basement membrane,
     mucociliary transport,
     innervation, etc.
- Circadian rhythm

- Triggers
  Indirect (cold air, smoke)
  Direct (pollen, animals)
- Patterns of inflammation
- Hyperresponsiveness
- Acute and late phase

---

symptoms are also more intense in patients with asthma than in patients with rhinitis alone.

Anatomic and Physiologic Similarities of Rhinitis and Asthma

There are many similarities between the upper and lower airways, including a continuous basement membrane, pseudostratified columnar epithelium, mucosal transport, tubuloalveolar seromucous glands, goblet cells, parasympathetic and sympathetic innervation, and circadian rhythm response (Table 9-2).

Triggers for upper and lower airway responsiveness are the same, including nonspecific irritants (e.g., cold air, cigarette smoke) and allergens, both seasonal (pollens and mold) and perennial (house dust mite and animals). The cellular mediators of inflammation for both include mast cells, eosinophils, basophils, and Th2 lymphocytes. The number of eosinophils in the nose has been shown to correlate with eosinophilic infiltration in the bronchi. Finally, both the nose and the lung demonstrate airway hyperresponsiveness as well as an acute and late phase response. In patients with pure rhinitis and no evidence of asthma, inhalation of methacholine, a parasympathomimetic agent, results in an increase in lower airway responsiveness that approaches that seen in asthma.

Changes in the Nose That Affect the Lower Airway

In addition to the horizontal relationship between rhinitis and asthma (i.e., the impressive co-existence of rhinitis and asthma), there is also a vertical relationship, by which changes in the nose affect the lower airway. One example is the important role the nose plays in warming and humidifying inspired air. If the nose is bypassed, then cold dry air reaches the lung. In one study on exercise-induced asthma, subjects with spontaneous breathing (i.e., breathing through both the nose and mouth) showed a slight decrease in FEV_1 compared with subjects with exclusive nasal breathing. Mouth breathers showed a much greater decline in FEV_1 with exercise.

Nasal provocation has also been shown to alter lower airway function. In patients with pure allergic rhinitis and no evidence of asthma, both clinically and by pulmonary function tests, stimulation of the nose by histamine resulted in a fall in FEV_1. If nasal allergen challenge is performed out of season in patients with both seasonal rhinitis and asthma, there is a marked increase in lower airway responsiveness.

Another example of the upper and lower airway relationship is that a viral upper respiratory tract infection (URI) is clearly the most important cause of emergency room visits and hospitalizations for asthma. During a viral URI, the lower airway is more responsive to both histamine and allergen inhalation.

Evidence for a nasal-bronchial reflex has been seen in studies on patients with unilateral trigeminal neuralgia who have a nerve resection performed. Brief nasal exposure to silica on both sides of the nose showed a significant increase in lower airway resistance after silica exposure on the intact side with no change seen on the resected side.

The Effect of Treatment of Rhinitis on Asthma

Many studies show that treatment of seasonal allergic rhinitis has beneficial effects on asthma. One of the first utilized intranasal corticosteroids in patients with both seasonal allergic rhinitis and asthma. While the expected result was an improvement in rhinitis symptoms, there was also a significant improvement seen in asthma scores (4). An inhibition of seasonal elevation in lower airway responsiveness and a reduction in exercise-induced bronchoconstriction has also been demonstrated with nasal corticosteroids. Similar beneficial effects on asthma have been seen with antihistamines and antihistamine-decongestant combinations. Finally, there is some evidence that immunotherapy for rhinitis will decrease the chances for the development of bronchial asthma.

Summary

There are many anatomic and physiologic similarities between the nose and the lungs. There is also extensive evidence that a decrease in nasal function adversely affects the lungs and that nasal provocation will alter lower airway function. There is ample evidence from clinical trials that treatment of rhinitis with either local or systemic agents will result in clinical and physiologic improvement of lower airway disease (Case 9-1).

Rhinosinusitis

It has been recently suggested that the term *sinusitis* be replaced by *rhinosinusitis,* a more descriptive and accurate word for the following reasons: Rhinitis typically precedes sinusitis, and sinusitis without rhinitis is rare; the mucosa of the nose and sinuses are contiguous, and symptoms of nasal obstruction and nasal discharge are prominent in sinusitis.

CASE 9-1 *Treatment of rhinitis resulting in improvement of asthma symptoms*

A 21-year-old college senior developed allergic rhinitis at age 12. Five years later, asthma began. He had been skin tested and reacted to tree pollen, ragweed pollen, and house dust mite. At the time of his initial evaluation, he was on no medications. He complained of dyspnea on exertion, nocturnal awakening with cough and wheeze, nasal congestion, and rhinorrhea. On physical examination, his nasal turbinates were swollen and pale; his chest examination revealed scattered expiratory wheezes. Pulmonary function tests showed an FEV_1 of 62% of predicted and an FEF_{25-75} of 48% of predicted.

The patient was started on an inhaled corticosteroid and a long-acting beta-agonist, both two puffs, twice a day. He returned one month later, feeling better with respect to his chest. He now awakened only twice per week with coughing and wheezing, and his exercise-induced asthma was still present but lessened. Nasal symptoms persisted. His chest was clear, and his nose still revealed swollen turbinates. Pulmonary function tests showed an FEV_1 of 75% of predicted and an FEF_{25-75} of 57% predicted. Asthma medications were continued, and a nasal corticosteroid was added. One month later, he was completely asymptomatic: FEV_1 was 88% of predicted and FEF_{25-75} was 74% of predicted.

Discussion

This patient had both allergic rhinitis and asthma. Appropriate asthma medications improved his condition, but it was not until his rhinitis was adequately treated that pulmonary function function tests returned to normal.

Rhinosinusitis is an extremely common disorder. It is the most frequently reported chronic disease in the United States, affecting 14.7% of the population. It accounts for 11.6 million physician office visits per year and for the fifth highest antibiotic use of all diseases.

The most important clinical clue to the diagnosis of acute rhinosinusitis is the failure of symptoms to resolve after a typical cold. The patient will note that the nasal discharge that had previously been clear becomes yellow or green. Fever persists, chills may develop, and pain more severe on bending or straining is often felt in the cheek. On physical examination, thick, purulent green or deep-yellow secretions are seen most often in the middle meatus, which is the draining site of the maxillary sinus.

If mucopus is not evacuated, then acute rhinosinusitis may enter a subacute or chronic phase. Here, the diagnostic index of suspicion of the physician must be high, for the typical clinical presentation of chronic rhinosinusitis is subtle. The patient generally presents with nasal stuffiness, purulent post-nasal drainage, sore throat, hyposmia, fetid breath, and malaise. On physical examination, an edematous and hyperemic nasal mucosa is generally bathed in mucopus. Nasal endoscopy may be useful for visualizing the middle meatus and the flow of infected mucus. In some instances, sinus imaging may be necessary to make the diagnosis of rhino-sinusitis. Coronal CT scan is the radiographic modality of choice.

The frequent association of paranasal sinus disease and bronchial asthma has been noted for many years. A number of clinical studies in the 1920s and 1930s emphasized the importance of sinusitis as a trigger for asthma. However, the relationship between sinusitis and asthma then seemed to fall into disrepute, and little was written about this relationship for the next several decades. One prevailing thought was that sinus changes simply reflected a disease of the entire respiratory membrane. Therefore management of rhinosinusitis *per se* would be expected to have little effect on the course of lower respiratory tract disease. In the last two decades, the relationship of rhinosinusitis and asthma has been revived.

Association of Rhinosinusitis and Asthma

There is no question that a high incidence of radiographic evidence of rhino-sinusitis is present in both children and adults with asthma. One recent study from Los Angeles Children's Hospital showed that 75% of pediatric patients admitted with status asthmaticus had abnormal sinus x-rays. An adult study from Finland reported abnormal sinus radiographs in 87% of patients with an exacerbation of asthma.

There has been a suggestion that the association between chronic rhino-sinusitis and asthma was strong only in the group of sinusitis patients with extensive disease. It appears that peripheral blood eosinophilia is a good marker for extensive rhinosinusitis. The overriding question is whether this association represents an epiphenomenona; that is: Are rhinosinusitis and asthma manifestations of the same underlying disease process in different parts of the respiratory tract, or is there a causal relationship? Can rhino-sinusitis trigger bronchial asthma?

Although more objective evidence is needed, there are data that indi-cate that difficult-to-control asthma will improve when co-existent rhino-sinusitis is cleared by medical and/or surgical treatment.

Nasal Polyposis

Nasal polyps appear to be outgrowths of the nasal mucosa and are typi-cally smooth, gelatinous, semitranslucent, round or pear-shaped, and pale. They are located on the lateral wall of the nose and rise mainly from the ethmoid sinus.

The association of nasal polyps and asthma has long been recognized. One large series of patients with nasal polyposis found an asthma incidence of 20%. In this same study, 32% of asthmatic patients had nasal polyps.

The association of nasal polyps, bronchial asthma, and aspirin sensitivity has been well described as the aspirin triad or Samter's triad. Vasomotor rhinitis associated with profuse rhinorrhea generally occurs first in these patients. Intense nasal congestion then follows with the subsequent development of nasal polyps. After this, bronchial asthma develops and, finally, aspirin sensitivity.

Results of Therapy of Rhinosinusitis on Asthma

There is no controlled study in adults demonstrating that medical therapy for rhinosinusitis improves asthma, although anecdotal evidence abounds. There are, however, a number of studies in children that show a significant improvement of the asthmatic state with appropriate antibiotic treatment for associated rhinosinusitis. In one study, 79% of the children were able to discontinue bronchodilator therapy after resolution of the rhinosinusitis. Pulmonary function tests showed normal results in 67% of those with pretreatment abnormalities.

We had an opportunity to observe a large group of adult patients with coexistent rhinosinusitis and asthma, who also presented with suggestive evidence that rhinosinusitis played an important role in the pathogenesis of their asthma. More than 90% gave a history indicating that their rhinosinusitis preceded the development of asthma symptoms. Based on history and a battery of allergy skin tests to common St. Louis aeroallergens, two-thirds of the patients were judged to be nonatopic, and more than 50% gave a history of aspirin sensitivity. Most importantly, more than 90% of these patients were receiving systemic corticosteroids for asthma control. Corticosteroid dependency furnishes an important clue to those patients in whom an underlying rhinosinusitis may act as a trigger for the development of asthma. These patients manifested rhinosinusitis that was uniformly medically resistant (i.e., rhinosinusitis either recurred or never sufficiently resolved with aggressive medical management).

Results obtained with bilateral intranasal sphenoethmoidectomy (BSE) showed that the asthma symptoms improved significantly in 65% of these patients. Patients who showed improvement within the 2 years following surgery were likely to experience continued improvement throughout a 5-year observation period. More than 80% of the patients reported that they had experienced moderately or greatly improved nasal symptoms, and 60% felt that asthma symptoms had improved. Prednisone requirements in the group fell from an average of 25 to 7.5 mg per day.

Equally good results have been obtained with a less radical operative procedure, functional endoscopic sinus surgery (FESS). One study reported results from a trial involving 205 adult patients with the "aspirin triad" (nasal polyps, asthma, and aspirin sensitivity), all of whom were steroid dependent (5). After FESS, 40% were able to discontinue steroids and another 44% were controlled on alternate-day or bursts of steroids. This is particularly notable because patients with the aspirin triad have asthma that is extremely difficult to control. Another study looked at 20 patients, aged 16 to 72 years old, with chronic rhinosinusitis and asthma (6). Following FESS, 70% reported

> **CASE 9-2   *Surgical treatment of rhinosinusitis resulting in improvement of asthma symptoms***
>
> A 57-year-old teacher developed asthma for the first time along with nasal congestion and purulent postnasal drainage. Examination of the chest revealed generalized rhonchi and wheezing. The nose showed swollen erythematous turbinates with mucopus in the nose and posterior pharynx. Chest radiograph showed hyperinflation. Sinus radiographs showed marked mucoperiosteal thickening and air fluid levels in the maxillary sinuses.
>
> Antibiotics were begun, along with oral decongestants and nasal steroids, resulting in a marked improvement in chest and nasal symptoms. In the next 6 months, despite appropriate antibiotic therapy, the patient developed four more sinus infections, each associated with exacerbation of asthma. Sinus CT showed pansinusitis. Functional endoscopic sinus surgery was performed with marked improvement in nasal, sinus, and chest symptoms, which continued over the next 4 years.
>
> **Discussion**
>
> Rhinosinusitis is frequently associated with asthma. When medical therapy fails, surgical intervention to correct the rhinosinusitis must be considered.

the frequency of asthma to be much less and 65% reported significantly less severe asthma. Of particular interest was a 75% reduction in hospitalization and an 81% reduction in emergency department/urgent office visits in the year following FESS.

Mechanisms Relating Rhinosinusitis to Asthma

Although a number of possibilities have been suggested, the precise mechanisms linking rhinosinusitis to asthma are not known. A recent theory proposes that the airway hyperresponsiveness seen in rhinosinusitis might depend on pharyngobronchial reflexes triggered by seeding of the inflammatory process into the pharynx through post-nasal drip of mediators and infected material from affected sinuses. The theory is based on the finding that intrabronchial and particularly extrabronchial reactivity were strongly associated with the degree of pharyngitis as determined by history, physical examination, and nasal lavage. In a later study, the authors demonstrated actual damage of pharyngeal mucosa in patients with chronic rhinosinusitis marked by epithelial thinning and a striking increase in pharyngeal nerve fiber density (7). This would favor increased access of irritants to submucosal nerve endings inducing the release of sensory neuropeptides via axon reflexes with activation of a neural arch, resulting in reflex airway constriction.

The diagnostic index of suspicion for rhinosinusitis must be high in any case of difficult-to-control asthma. While the precise mechanism is not known, there are enough clinical data to strongly link rhinosinusitis with asthma. Appropriate medical and/or surgical therapy of underlying rhinosinusitis will frequently result in improvement in the associated asthma (Case 9-2).

Summary

There appear to be important links between the upper and lower airways. Physicians must become accustomed to examining both parts of the respiratory tract. Patients with rhinitis should be observed carefully for the development of asthma, and those with asthma should be considered to have either rhinitis or rhinosinusitis. Attention to both the nose and sinuses will frequently benefit asthma.

■   ■   ■

Key Points

- More than half of patients with rhinitis have asthma, and most (up to 95%) patients with asthma have rhinitis.

- Both allergic and nonalllergic rhinitis are strongly associated with asthma, with rhinitis serving as a risk factor for asthma and worsening its severity.

- Changes in the nose (e.g., the warming and humidifying of inspired air) affect lower airway function.

- Clinical trials have shown that treatment of rhinitis with local or systemic agents results in improvement of lower airway disease.

- Sinusitis is a frequent precipitator of asthma, and medical or surgical treatment of the underlying sinusitis will often benefit the asthmatic state.

■   ■   ■

REFERENCES

1. **Togias AG.** Systemic immunologic and inflammatory aspects of allergic rhinitis. J Allergy Clin Immunol. 2000;106:S247–50.

2. **Leynaert B, Neukvich F, Demoly P, Bousquet J.** Epidemiologic evidence for asthma and rhinitis comorbidity. J Allergy Clin Immunol. 2000;106:S201–5.

3. **Greisner WA III, Settipane RJ, Settipane GA.** Co-existence of asthma and allergic rhinitis: a 23-year follow-up study of college students. Allergy Asthma Proc. 1998;19:185–8.

4. **Welsh PW, Stricker WE, Chu CP, et al.** Efficacy of beclomethasone nasal solution, flunisolide and cromolyn in relieving symptoms of ragweed allergy. Mayo Clin Proc. 1987;62:125–34.

5. **English GM.** Nasal polypectomy and sinus surgery in patients with asthma and aspirin idiosyncrasy. Laryngoscope. 1986;96:374–80.

6. **Nishioka GJ, Cook PR, Davies WE, et al.** Functional endoscopic sinus surgery in patients with chronic sinusitis and asthma. Otolarngol Head Neck Surg. 1994;110:494–500.

7. **Rolla G, Cologrand P, Scappaticci E, et al.** Damage of the pharyngeal mucosa and hyperresponsiveness of the airway in sinusitis. J Allergy Clin Immunol. 1997;100:52–7.

SUGGESTED READING

Simons FER. Allergic rhinobronchitis: the asthma-allergic rhinitis link. J Allergy Clin Immunol. 1999;104:534–40.

10

■ ■ ■

Asthma During Pregnancy

Michael Schatz, MD, MS

A sthma is one of the most common potentially serious medical problems in pregnancy. The incidence of asthma in pregnant women in older retrospective studies was 1%, but recent prevalence data suggest an incidence of up to 7%. Managing asthma during pregnancy is unique because the effect of both the illness and treatment on the developing fetus and patient must be considered. In addition, pregnancy may alter the course of asthma. After reviewing respiratory physiology during pregnancy, this chapter discusses the relationships between asthma and pregnancy, nonpharmacologic management of gestational asthma, general and specific aspects of pharmacologic therapy during pregnancy, and obstetric management of the pregnant asthmatic patient.

Respiratory Physiology During Pregnancy

Maternal Physiology

Minute ventilation increases during pregnancy, presumably due to increased circulating levels of progesterone. The increased minute ventilation exceeds metabolic demands and results in a compensated respiratory alkalosis during pregnancy. Thus normal blood gases during pregnancy reveal a higher pO_2 (100 to 106 mm Hg) and a lower pCO_2 (28 to 30 mm Hg) than in the nonpregnant state.

Two major consequences of this pregnancy-induced hyperventilation are specifically relevant to women with asthma. First, the changes in blood gases that occur secondary to acute asthma during pregnancy will be superimposed on the "normal" respiratory alkalosis of pregnancy. Thus a $pCO_2 > 35$ or a $pO_2 < 70$ associated with acute asthma will represent more severe compromise during pregnancy than will similar blood gases in the nongravid state. Second, the hyperventilation of pregnancy appears to be related to the dyspnea of early pregnancy seen in up to 60% to 75% of pregnant women. This dyspnea, which most frequently begins in the first or second trimester, as well as the dyspnea apparently caused by upward pressure on the diaphragm near term, must be differentiated from dyspnea caused by asthma. However, because these dyspneas of pregnancy are not associated with wheezing or cough, this differentiation is usually not difficult for physicians or patients.

Several lung volume changes occur during pregnancy. Tidal volume increases during pregnancy, whereas residual volume and functional residual capacity (FRC) decrease. In spite of reduced FRC during pregnancy, vital capacity and total lung capacity are usually preserved due to unimpaired diaphragmatic excursion and the increased mobility and flaring of the ribs during pregnancy. This decrease in FRC means that airway closure may be more likely to occur with tidal breathing during pregnancy, especially in the supine position. This effect may lead to decreased ventilation to certain parts of the lung and potential ventilation-perfusion imbalance. Although these changes do not generally affect normal pregnancy, they may intensify the low ventilation/perfusion ratios and the resting hypoxemia that occur secondary to bronchial obstruction when acute asthma complicates pregnancy. One practical implication of this information is that women with acute asthma during pregnancy should maintain the seated rather than the supine position.

Airway mechanics do not change significantly during pregnancy. Thus no changes in forced expiratory volume in one second (FEV_1), FEV_1/FVC ratio, or maximum mid-expiratory flow rates (MMEF) have been reported during pregnancy. One study suggested that peak expiratory flow rate and FEV_1 are lower during pregnancy in the supine compared with the seated position, again reinforcing the advantages of the latter position for women with symptomatic gestational asthma.

Fetal Physiology

Fetal oxygenation and monitoring have been recently reviewed (1). Arterial pO_2 in the fetus is only about one-third to one-fourth the arterial pO_2 in the adult. This is because the human placenta acts as a simple concurrent exchanger and because fetal umbilical vein blood leaving the placenta exists in oxygen equilibrium with maternal uterine vein blood. Thus fetal umbilical vein blood has the highest fetal pO_2 and can never exceed maternal venous pO_2. The fetus normally thrives at this low oxygen level due to a number of compensations; however, fetal oxygenation may be threatened in a number of ways potentially relevant to gestational asthma. First, maternal hypoxia directly reduces oxygen supply to the fetus. Second, hypocapnia and/or alkalosis itself apparently may cause fetal hypoxia, although the exact mechanism is unclear. Finally, reduction in uterine blood flow (potentially due to exogenous or endogenous vasoconstrictors, dehydration, or significant maternal alkalosis) may compromise fetal oxygenation.

It does appear that the fetus can compensate for hypoxia in a number of ways, including redistribution of circulation to vital organs, decreased gross body movements, and increased tissue oxygen extraction. The exact level and duration of fetal hypoxia that exceeds its ability to compensate is not defined in humans. A common response to chronic hypoxia is deferment of growth needs in favor of vital functions, resulting in a small-for-gestational-age fetus.

Relationships Between Asthma and Pregnancy

Effect of Asthma on Mother and Fetus

Epidemiologic Studies
Controlled studies that have evaluated outcomes of pregnancy in asthmatic compared with nonasthmatic women have been recently reviewed (2). A meta-analysis of these studies reported a statistically significant increased risk in the pregnancies of asthmatic versus nonasthmatic women of perinatal mortality, preeclampsia, low birth weight infants, and preterm births, but not congenital malformations. A more recent study (3) described the outcomes of pregnancy in 36,985 women identified as having asthma in either the Swedish Medical Birth Registry and/or the Swedish Hospital Discharge Registry. These outcomes were compared with the total of 1.32 million births that occurred in the Swedish population during the years of the study (1984-1995). The results were qualitatively similar to those of the aforementioned meta-analysis. Both the meta-analysis and the Swedish study suggested that patients with more severe asthma were at greater risk. In the meta-analysis, studies in which oral steroids were required by a higher proportion of patients generally reported greater risks compared with studies in which steroid treatment was less frequent. In the Swedish study, patients identified as having asthma by both the hospital discharge registry and the medical birth registry, who would presumably be more definite and more severe asthmatics, manifested higher risks than all asthmatic patients identified.

The literature also contains case reports of perinatal mortality associated with severe uncontrolled asthma (2). In addition, two studies have reported an increased incidence of transient tachypnea of the neonate and neonatal hyperbilirubinemia in infants of asthmatic versus control mothers (2).

In addition to fetal morbidity and mortality, severe asthma during pregnancy may be a cause of maternal mortality (2). Three studies have reported increased incidences of antepartum hemorrhage and cesarean section in asthmatic gravidas compared with control gravidas (2).

Mechanisms

Definition of the mechanism(s) of maternal asthma's adverse effect on pregnancy should allow institution of optimal intervention strategy. Mechanisms postulated to explain the possible increased perinatal risks have included 1) hypoxia and other physiologic consequences of poorly controlled asthma, 2) medications used to treat asthma, and 3) demographic or pathogenic factors *associated with* asthma but actually not caused by the disease or its treatment. Data supporting specific mechanisms for the most common specific adverse outcomes have been recently reviewed (2,4). Although demographic factors more prevalent in asthmatic subjects (e.g., smoking, African American race) could account for some of the excess adverse outcomes, increased risks persisted in studies that controlled for these confounding factors. The published data do not fully define the mechanism(s) of maternal asthma's potential adverse effects on pregnancy and the infant. Available information, however, suggests that poor asthma control may be the most remedial factor and supports the important generalization that adequate asthma control during pregnancy is important in improving maternal/fetal outcome. In accord with this hypothesis is the observation that studies in which the gestational asthma has been managed by specialists do not report increased adverse fetal outcomes in infants of asthmatic women compared with control infants (4).

Effect of Pregnancy on Asthma

Epidemiology

Fourteen studies have evaluated the change in asthma course during pregnancy. The sample size in these studies varied from 16 to 366, and the variation in results was equally large. Improvement in asthma course occurred in 0% to 69% of patients, worsening of asthma in 0% to 44%, and no change in asthma severity in 6% to 100% (4). There are at least two likely reasons for this variability: 1) the method by which asthma course during pregnancy was assessed, and 2) the asthma severity of the population being studied, since review of the data suggests that asthmatic women with more severe asthma before becoming pregnant are more likely to deteriorate during pregnancy. The commonly quoted generalization is that during pregnancy, about one-third of patients with asthma experience improvement of symptoms, one-third experience worsening of symptoms, and one-third remain the same. A meta-analysis of these fourteen studies agreed with this generalization (4).

The course of asthma may vary by stage of pregnancy (4). The first trimester is generally well-tolerated in asthmatics with infrequent acute episodes. Increased symptoms and more frequent exacerbations have been reported to occur between weeks 17 and 36 of gestation (Case 10-1). In contrast, asthmatic women in general tend to experience fewer symptoms and less frequent asthma exacerbations during weeks 37 to 40 of

CASE 10-1 *Patient with acute asthma during the third trimester of pregnancy*

A 32-year-old gravida I para 0 woman presents in her seventh month of pregnancy with increasing asthma symptoms. She has had asthma since childhood, but it has been worsening since she has been pregnant. Previous allergy evaluation revealed negative allergy skin tests. She has been taking salmeterol 2 puffs bid, budesonide 2 puffs bid, and inhaled albuterol as needed. She was not having daily symptoms or interference with sleep due to asthma until the onset of a cold 6 days earlier. The cold is improving, she denies purulent mucus, but her asthma is now keeping her from sleeping, and she is using her albuterol inhaler every 3 hr. Her personal best peak flow is 420, but her peak flow this morning was 210. She denies edema or any other significant medical history.

Examination reveals a woman in mild respiratory distress with diffuse expiratory wheezing. Her pulse was 102, BP 150/90, oxygen saturation 96%, and FEV_1 50% of predicted. After 4 puffs of inhaled albuterol with a spacer, she was no longer in respiratory distress and her FEV_1 improved to 65% of predicted, but her BP remained somewhat elevated (145/85).

Discussion

Recommendations for this patient were as follows: 1) prednisone 40 mg daily for 3 days, then call physician with a progress report; 2) a return asthma appointment in 1 week; and 3) an urgent obstetrics appointment for evaluation of possible pregnancy-induced hypertension.

pregnancy than during any prior 4-week gestational period. Even patients who had overall worsening of asthma during pregnancy in one study experienced statistically significant improvement during their last month of pregnancy (4). These studies suggest that the first trimester and the last month of pregnancy are relatively free of asthma exacerbations and that the second and earlier third trimester have more potential for increased asthma symptoms.

Finally, asthma generally remains quiescent during labor and delivery itself. Ninety percent of 360 asthmatic women in one study had no symptoms of asthma at all during labor and delivery (4). Of the ones who did, approximately half required no acute treatment, some used inhaled bronchodilators, and only two required intravenous aminophylline.

Mechanisms

The variable effect of pregnancy on the course of asthma appears to be more than just random fluctuation in the natural history of the disease, since the changes in asthma course that women attribute to pregnancy generally revert toward the pre-pregnancy course in the 3 months postpartum (4). It is also of interest that the course of asthma is often consistent in an individual woman during successive pregnancies (4).

Table 10-1   Physiologic Changes During Pregnancy That May Affect the Course of Asthma

Physiologic Change	Effect on Asthma
Factors That May Improve Asthma	
Increased progesterone	Direct bronchodilation or potentiation of β–adrenergic bronchodilation
Increased estrogen	Potentiation of β–adrenergic bronchodilation
Decreased plasma histamine	Decreased histamine-mediated brochoconstriction
Increased serum free cortisol	Direct pulmonary effects of corticosteroids or corticosteroid-mediated increased β–adrenergic responsiveness
Increased serum prostagandin E	Brochodilation
Increased prostaglandin I_2	Bronchial stabilization
Increased serum atrial natriuretic factor	Bronchodilation
Pharmacokinetic changes	Increased half-life or decreased protein binding of endogenous or exogenous bronchodilators
Factors That May Worsen Asthma	
Increased progesterone, aldosterone, and deoxycorticosterone	Pulmonary refractoriness to cortisol because of competitive binding to glucocorticosteroid receptors
Increased serum prostaglandin $F_{2\alpha}$	Bronchconstriction
Decreased functional residual capacity	Airway closure during tidal breathing and altered ventilation-perfusion ratios
Increased placental major basic protein	Adverse pulmonary effects
Increased gastroesphageal reflux	Asthma aggravation

The mechanisms responsible for the altered asthma course during pregnancy are unknown and represent a fertile area for additional research. Many biochemical and physiological changes during pregnancy could potentially ameliorate or exacerbate gestational asthma (Table 10-1). However, it is not clear which, if any, of these factors are actually important in determining asthma course during pregnancy.

Additional factors may contribute to asthma course during pregnancy. Pregnancy may be a source of stress for many women, and this stress could aggravate asthma. Adherence to medication can change during pregnancy, with a corresponding change in asthma control. Most commonly observed is decreased adherence due to a mother's concerns about the safety of medication for the fetus.

Physician reluctance to treat may also affect asthma severity during pregnancy. A recent surveillance study identified 51 pregnant women and

500 nonpregnant women presenting to the emergency department with acute asthma (5). Although asthma severity appeared to be similar in the two groups based on peak flow rates, pregnant women were significantly less likely to be treated with systemic steroids in the emergency department (44% vs. 66%) and significantly less likely to be discharged on oral steroids (38% vs. 64%). Presumably related to this undertreatment, pregnant women were three times more likely than nonpregnant women to report an ongoing exacerbation 2 weeks later ($P = 0.02$).

The fetus itself could affect asthma course during pregnancy. It has been hypothesized that fetal antigenicity could lead to an immunological response that might exacerbate asthma. In addition, the gender of the fetus may play a role. A recent small prospective study, in which women rated their gestational asthma severity before they knew the gender of their baby, reported that women carrying female fetuses described significantly more severe symptoms than those carrying male fetuses. A surge of androgens produced by male fetuses at 12 to 16 weeks was suggested as a possible explanation.

Infections during pregnancy may certainly affect the course of gestational asthma. Some degree of decrease in cell-mediated immunity may make the pregnant patient more susceptible to viral infections, and upper respiratory tract infections have been reported to be the most common precipitants of severe asthma during pregnancy (4). Sinusitis, a known asthma trigger, has been shown to be six times more common in pregnant compared with nonpregnant women. In addition, pneumonia has been reported to be more than five times more common in asthmatic women than in nonasthmatic women during pregnancy.

Finally, changes in specific IgE or environmental exposure may influence gestational asthma course. Most pregnant asthmatic patients appear to be atopic. In one study, pregnant atopic patients were reported to manifest milder asthma with fewer hospitalizations than nonatopic patients. In contrast, a positive correlation between levels of specific IgE against cockroach antigen and gestational asthma severity was recently described in pregnant inner-city women. Further studies will be necessary to clarify the relationships between atopy, environmental exposures, pregnancy, and asthma course.

Asthma Management During Pregnancy

Goals of Therapy

Two main goals of asthma management appear appropriate to optimize both maternal and fetal health. Prevention of acute episodes should prevent potentially harmful acute hypoxia, hypocapnia, alkalosis, and dehydration. Optimization of chronic maternal pulmonary function should reduce the potential for chronic hypoxia and maternal symptoms as well as the likelihood of acute episodes.

Nonpharmacologic Management

The identification of potentially avoidable triggering factors is an important aspect of nonpharmacologic management that may prevent acute episodes, improve clinical well-being, and decrease the need for pharmacologic intervention. It is particularly important for the pregnant asthmatic woman to discontinue smoking during pregnancy. First, smoking may predispose to increased asthma, complicating bronchitis or sinusitis and thus increasing the need for medication. Second, the increased perinatal morbidity attributed to smoking may be additive to that conferred by uncontrolled maternal asthma (4).

Historical information or previous skin testing will often suggest mite, mold, dander, or pollen sensitivity for which avoidance may be advised. Routine skin testing in previously untested patients is usually deferred in our clinic until postpartum, since skin testing with potent antigens may be associated with systemic reactions. *In vitro* tests for specific IgE may be obtained if confirmation of historically relevant allergens is necessary during pregnancy.

Spontaneous abortions associated with systemic reactions following allergen immunotherapy have been reported. In addition, anaphylaxis due to other causes has been associated with maternal and fetal mortality and morbidity. Aside from systemic reactions, allergy immunotherapy appears safe during pregnancy. Two studies of 121 pregnancies in 90 women and 109 pregnancies in 81 women receiving inhalant allergen immunotherapy reported no increase in abortions, perinatal deaths, prematurity, toxemia, or congenital malformations in the treated patients compared with both a nontreated pregnant allergic control group and the general population.

Based on this information, it is recommended that allergen immunotherapy be continued carefully during pregnancy in patients already receiving it who appear to be deriving benefit, who are not prone to systemic reactions, and who are receiving a maintenance or at least a substantial dosage. Dose reduction is recommended to decrease the risk of a systemic reaction; similarly, it is usually appropriate to discontinue immunotherapy in patients who would require further increases to achieve therapeutic doses. Benefit-risk considerations do not favor beginning immunotherapy during pregnancy for most patients due to the

1. Undefined propensity for systemic reactions
2. Increased likelihood of systemic reactions during initiation of immunotherapy
3. Latency of the immunotherapy effect
4. Frequent difficulty in predicting which asthmatic patients will benefit from immunotherapy

As mentioned previously, asthma may add to the stress of normal pregnancy and, conversely, this stress may aggravate asthma. It is important that anxiety in pregnant patients be reduced by giving patients the opportunity to express their concerns and educating them regarding their illness and its interactions with pregnancy. Educational material for pregnant asthmatic patients has been published (6). Such education should also improve patient adherence.

Careful follow-up by physicians experienced in managing asthma is an essential aspect of optimal gestational asthma management. Asthmatic women requiring regular medication should be evaluated at least monthly. In addition to symptomatic and auscultatory assessment, objective measures of respiratory status (optimally spirometry, minimally PEF) should be obtained at every visit. In addition, patients with more severe or labile asthma should be considered for home PEF monitoring. All pregnant patients should have ready access to their physician when symptoms increase. It is also important that effective communication exists among the physician managing the asthma, the patient, and the obstetrician

Pharmacologic Management

General Considerations
Medication during pregnancy may have several types of adverse effects on the fetus or the pregnancy:

1. Abortion
2. Fetal death
3. Congenital malformation (especially first trimester exposure)
4. Effect on fetal growth
5. Effect on function of developing organs (e.g., the central nervous system)
6. Effect on maternal or uteroplacental vasculature or uterine smooth muscle
7. Effect of transplacentally administered drugs in the newborn

Although few drugs have been proven harmful, and fewer than 1% of congenital malformations can be attributed to drugs, statistical and ethical considerations make it unlikely that any drug will ever be "proven safe." Although unnecessary use of medication during pregnancy should be avoided, the potential risks of untreated disease make pharmacologic intervention for gestational asthma often necessary.

The choice of a specific medication for use during pregnancy is based on a number of considerations:

Human Data—Human data exist in the form of case reports, cohort studies, and case-control studies. Case reports, in which an exposure and an outcome are presented, should not be used to infer cause and effect. Cohort studies prospectively evaluate exposed and nonexposed populations to determine outcome, and case-control studies retrospectively evaluate affected and nonaffected subjects for whether or not they were exposed. Negative cohort studies are reassuring but rarely include sufficient numbers of exposed individuals to rule out a small (but important) increase in adverse pregnancy outcome, especially when dealing with outcomes such as specific malformations, the most common of which may only occur in 3 per 1000 births. Positive cohort or case-control studies do not of themselves prove causation and generally must be considered to suggest hypotheses requiring independent confirmation. Nonetheless, when effective alternatives are available, it seems advisable to avoid drugs implicated in cohort or case-control studies.

2. *Animal Data*—Although animals differ from humans in a number of ways, animal teratology experiments can be useful in evaluating human drug risks. Animal studies are designed to maximize the response of the system to potential toxic effects of the test agent by using large doses. It is believed that a testing scheme using appropriate doses in at least two species, one of which is a nonrodent, is sufficient to raise suspicion of human developmental risk. There are, in fact, no known human developmental toxicants that would not have been identified in this manner. Thus, if an agent is appropriately tested in animals and found not to be a developmental toxicant, its potential for human developmental toxicity is low. Positive data in animal studies are not as useful, because it is often not possible to know whether species differences, the clinically irrelevant high doses used, or maternal toxicity is responsible for the adverse effects on the offspring.

3. *FDA Categories*—In 1979, the United States Food and Drug Administration established five categories to describe a drug's potential for causing adverse effects during pregnancy (Table 10-2) and mandated that newly approved drugs introduced after 1 November 1980 be classified into one of these categories in the package insert. The categories are based on the results

Table 10-2   Food and Drug Administration Pregnancy Categories

Category	Animal Studies	Human Data	Benefit May Outweigh Risk
A	Negative*	Studies† negative	Yes
B	Negative	Studies not done	Yes
B	Positive‡	Studies negative	Yes
C	Positive	Studies not done	Yes
C	Not done	Studies not done	Yes
D	Positive or negative	Studies or reports positive	Yes
X§	Positive	Studies or reports positive	No

* No teratogenicity demonstrated.
† Adequate and well-controlled studies in pregnant women.
‡ Teratogenicity demonstrated.
§ Drug contraindicated in pregnancy.

of animal studies, human data, and consideration of whether the benefit of the drug's use during pregnancy outweighs the risk. No asthma or allergy medication labeled to date meets the requirements for category A. One may wish to choose class B versus C drugs among equally effective alternatives due to the reassuring animal studies. Over the years, increasing dissatisfaction has arisen regarding the clinical usefulness of these categories, and the FDA is currently developing a new, more descriptive, system of pregnancy labeling.

4. *Other Considerations*—A topical medication would appear to be preferable to a systemic one due to reduced likelihood of fetal penetration. An older medication with a "track record" may be preferable to a newer one. Finally, absolute and relative efficacy must also be considered in the choice of a medication for use during pregnancy.

Specific Medications

Cohort studies have been reassuring regarding a lack of adverse effects on human pregnancy outcomes of metaproterenol, albuterol, theophylline, cromolyn, beclomethasone, and budesonide (7). In contrast, data regarding the use of oral corticosteroids during pregnancy have not been totally reassuring. Although cohort studies have not identified an increased risk of total malformations in the offspring of oral corticosteroid-treated mothers, three of four case-control studies have revealed a significantly increased risk of oral clefts in infants of corticosteroid-treated mothers.

Other adverse outcomes have also been attributed to oral corticosteroids, including an increased risk of preeclampsia, preterm birth, and lower birth weight (7). In many of these studies, it is difficult to exclude an adverse effect of the underlying disease itself. Moreover, authors of most of the foregoing studies have pointed out that these potential gestational risks of oral corticosteroids must be balanced against the risks to the mother or the infant of inadequately treated disease. In the case of asthma, as described above, the risks of severe uncontrolled asthma (which may include maternal or fetal mortality) would usually be the greater risk, which suggests that oral corticosteroids must still be used when indicated for the management of severe gestational asthma.

No human data exist for a number of newer medications currently used for asthma. These include drugs with reassuring animal studies (ipratropium, nedocromil, zafirlukast, and montelukast) and those with nonreassuring animal studies (salmeterol, zileuton). Recommendations for the use of these newer medications, based on the animal studies, route of administration, and efficacy considerations, are provided below.

Treatment Protocols

In 1993, the National Asthma Education Program Working Group on Asthma and Pregnancy published consensus recommendations for the management of gestational asthma (8). In 2000, these recommendations were updated by a joint *ad hoc* committee of the American College of Allergy, Asthma and Immunology (ACAAI) and the American College of Obstetricians and Gynecologists (ACOG) (9).

Chronic Asthma

The consensus recommendations for the management of chronic asthma during pregnancy are shown in Table 10-3. They are similar to the step therapy recommended for nonpregnant asthmatic patients, with a few exceptions. Although no recommendations regarding a specific inhaled beta-agonist were made in either of the aforementioned reports, the data reviewed above would suggest that metaproterenol or albuterol would be good choices. Because more published gestational human data exist for beclomethasone and budesonide, these were recommended if inhaled corticosteroids were being initiated during pregnancy (Case 10-2). The Working Group did recommend that other inhaled corticosteroids could be continued if the patient was well controlled on one of these medications before pregnancy, given the overall similarities in the systemic side effect profiles of currently available inhaled steroids at therapeutically equivalent doses and the likelihood that adverse effects may be a class effect. However, the FDA has recently approved a change in pregnancy classification for budesonide from Category C to Category B, based on controlled observational data from

Table 10-3   ACAAI-ACOG Recommendations for the Pharmacologic Step Therapy of Chronic Asthma During Pregnancy*

Category	Step Therapy
Mild intermittent	Inhaled β_2-agonists as needed (for all categories)[†]
Mild persistent	Inhaled cromolyn
	Continue inhaled nedocromil in patients who have shown a good response prior to pregnancy
	Substitute inhaled corticosteroids[‡] if above not adequate
Moderate persistent	Inhaled corticosteroid[‡]
	Continue inhaled salmeterol in patients who have shown a very good response prior to pregnancy
	Add oral theophylline and/or inhaled salmeterol for patients inadequately controlled by medium-dose inhaled corticosteroids
Severe persistent	Above + oral corticosteroids (burst for active symptoms, alternate-day or daily if necessary)

* Based on the recommendations of the National Asthma Education Program Report of the Working Group on Asthma During Pregnancy (8), updated to incorporate newer information (9).
† Most published human data study albuterol, metaproterenol, or terbutaline.
‡ Beclomethasone or budesonide if inhaled corticosteroids are being initiated during pregnancy; continuation of other inhaled corticosteroid if patient well-controlled by it before pregnancy; consider budesonide if patient requires high-dose inhaled corticosteroids for adequate control.

> **CASE 10-2**   *Patient with chronic asthma during the first trimester of pregnancy*
>
> A 23-year-old gravida II para I female presents during her first trimester of pregnancy with a history of asthma. She has not been hospitalized for asthma but did require an emergency department visit 6 months previously. Her asthma appeared to be worse during her previous pregnancy 2 years ago. She is now having daily symptoms and interference with sleep twice per week, and she is using her albuterol inhaler 3 or 4 times daily. She was given an inhaled corticosteroid inhaler 3 months ago but has been afraid to use it since she found out she was pregnant. She has noticed that cleaning house triggers her asthma. She has had a cat at home for 1 year (which she does not think aggravates her asthma) and does not smoke cigarettes. She has not been previously evaluated for allergies and denies any other significant medical history.
>
> Examination was unremarkable except for scattered end-expiratory wheezes. FEV_1 was 75% of predicted, which improved to 88% of predicted after 2 puffs of inhaled albuterol. The impression was moderate persistent asthma with a possible allergy component.
>
> **Discussion**
>
> Treatment for this patient was as follows: 1) education on asthma in general and asthma and pregnancy in particular; 2) allergy evaluation, especially for cat and mite allergy, and environmental control depending on the results; 3) beclomethasone or budesonide, with instructions on inhaler technique, 4) define her personal best peak flow rate and develop a peak flow-based action plan; and 5) follow-up in 2 to 4 weeks, then at least monthly during pregnancy, with facilitated access for increased problems between scheduled visits.

the Swedish Medical Birth Registry (7,9). Thus, because budesonide is now the only inhaled steroid with a Category B pregnancy classification, it may be most appropriate to use budesonide in all patients who need inhaled steroids during pregnancy. Avoidance of zileuton was recommended, but montelukast or zafirlukast may be considered for patients with recalcitrant asthma who had shown a uniquely favorable response before pregnancy. Salmeterol was recommended for pregnant asthmatics in the aforementioned Position Paper (9) for the following reasons: 1) the inhalation route for salmeterol makes the nonreassuring animal studies that used parenteral exposure less clinically relevant; 2) the chemical relationship between salmeterol and albuterol (for which there are reassuring animal data) provides reassurance; and 3) there exists a documented effect of salmeterol in patients not controlled on inhaled steroids.

Acute Asthma
The recommended therapy of acute asthma during pregnancy does not differ substantially from the management in nonpregnant patients (see

Chapter 4). Intensive fetal monitoring as well as maternal monitoring is essential. In addition to pharmacologic therapy, supplemental oxygen (initially 3 to 4 L/min by nasal cannula) should be administered, adjusting FiO_2 to maintain at $pO_2 \geq 70$ and/or O_2 saturation by pulse oximetry > 95%. Intravenous fluids (containing glucose if the patient is not hyperglycemic) should also be administered, initially at a rate of at least 100 mL/hr.

There are no data on the pharmacokinetics of exogenous corticosteroids administered during pregnancy, and dosages of corticosteroids recommended for pregnancy are generally not different than those recommended for nonpregnant patients. If intravenous aminophylline is used, pharmacokinetic studies during pregnancy suggest that the loading dose recommendation for theophylline requires no modification during pregnancy (5 mg/kg over 20 to 30 min), but the initial maintenance dose should be lower (0.5 mg/kg/hr). Studies have also suggested that protein binding of theophylline decreases during pregnancy such that there is an approximately 15% increase in free drug for any total drug concentration. This suggests that a lower therapeutic range (8 to 12 µg/mL) than usually recommended is appropriate during pregnancy. Because recent studies suggest that intravenous magnesium sulfate (1.0 to 2.0 g) may be beneficial in acute severe asthma as an adjunct to inhaled beta-agonists and intravenous corticosteroids, magnesium sulfate may also be considered, especially in patients with coexistent hypertension or preterm uterine contractions.

Intravenous cefuroxime is recommended initially for hospitalized pregnant asthmatic patients with suspected bacterial respiratory infections. Erythromycin should be included as part of initial therapy if *Mycoplasma pneumoniae*, *Chlamydia pneumoniae,* or *Legionella* infection is suspected.

Obstetric Management of Pregnant Asthmatic Patients

Detailed obstetric management of the pregnant asthmatic is described elsewhere (1). A number of medications potentially used for obstetric indications should be avoided in patients with asthma because they have been shown to trigger bronchospasm. These include beta-blockers, 15 methylprostaglandin $F_{2\alpha}$, transcervical or intra-amniotic prostaglandin E_2, methylergonovine or ergonovine, and nonsteroidal anti-inflammatory agents (in aspirin-sensitive asthmatics). Use of intravaginal or intracervical prostaglandin E_2 gel for cervical ripening before labor induction or prostaglandin E_2 suppositories for induced abortion or labor induction with a dead fetus has not been reported to cause bronchospasm in asthmatic patients. Magnesium sulfate and calcium-channel blockers, which have been shown to possess bronchodilator properties, should also be well-tolerated in asthmatic subjects.

Obstetric management during labor and delivery of women with controlled asthma is identical to management in nonasthmatic women, including the preference for regional versus general anesthesia. When general anesthesia is required for cesarean section, the following medications are recommended in asthmatic women because of their bronchodilating properties: 1) preanesthetic use of atropine and glycopyrrolate, 2) induction of anesthesia with ketamine, and 3) low concentrations of halogenated anesthetics.

Although only 10% of prospectively managed asthmatic women experience symptoms of asthma during labor or delivery, prophylactic medications should be continued. Patients experiencing asthma symptoms during labor should be treated with inhaled beta-agonists and parenteral corticosteroids if needed. For patients on regular corticosteroids or who have received frequent courses during pregnancy, supplemental corticosteroids for the stress of labor and delivery are recommended: 100 mg of hydrocortisone intravenously at admission followed by 100 mg intravenously every 8 hr for 24 hr or until the absence of complications is established.

Final Considerations

Managing asthma during pregnancy can be as satisfying as it is challenging. In our litigation-oriented society, however, the medicolegal implications of treating asthma during pregnancy must be considered. A number of steps have been recommended to reduce medicolegal jeopardy in managing gestational asthma:

1. Discuss with the patient the fact that, while relatively few medications of any kind have been "proven" harmful during pregnancy, no asthma/allergy medication can be considered "proven" absolutely safe.

2. Discuss the potential direct and indirect consequences for the mother and for the baby of inadequately controlled asthma.

3. Discuss the concept that there are medications that appear safe enough that their use is preferable to the uncontrolled illness that would result if they were not used.

4. Discuss the various medications available for the patient's particular situation and the rationale for choosing among those alternatives.

5. A written informed consent document is not recommended. However, clearly document in the chart that the foregoing discussion has taken place (i.e., the benefits, risks, and alternatives of the specific pharmacologic approach have been discussed with the patient, and her informed consent to that approach has been obtained).

REFERENCES

1. **Cousins L.** Fetal oxygenation, assessment of fetal well-being, and obstetric management of the pregnant patient with asthma. J Allergy Clin Immunol. 1999;103:S343–9.

2. **Schatz M, Dombrowski M.** Outcomes of pregnancy in asthmatic women. Immunol Allergy Clin N Amer. 2000;20:715–27.

3. **Kallen B, Rydhstroem H, Aberg A.** Asthma during pregnancy: a population-based study. Eur J Epidem. 2000;16:167–71.

4. **Schatz M.** Interrelationships between asthma and pregnancy: a literature review. J Allergy Clin Immunol. 1999;103:S330–6.

5. **Cydulka RK, Emerman CL, Schreiber D, et al.** Acute asthma among pregnant women presenting to the emergency department. Am J Respir Crit Care Med. 1999; 60:887–92.

6. **Lipkowitz MA, Schatz M, Cook TJ, et al.** Advice from your allergist: when allergies and asthma complicate pregnancy. Ann Allergy Asthma Immunol. 1998;81:30–4.

7. **Schatz M.** The efficacy and safety of asthma medications during pregnancy. Semin Perinatol. 2001;25:145–52.

8. **National Asthma Education Program.** Management of asthma during pregnancy: Report of the Working Group on Asthma and Pregnancy. NIH Publication No. 93-3279. Bethesda, MD: National Institutes of Health; 1993.

9. The use of newer asthma and allergy medications during pregnancy [Position Paper]. Ann Allergy Asthma Immunol. 2000;84:475–80.

SUGGESTED READING

Schatz M, ed. Asthma and allergy during pregnancy. Immunol Allergy Clin N Amer. 2000;20:663-878

11

∎ ∎ ∎

Asthma in the Elderly

Anthony Montanaro, MD

As we enter the new millennium, the demographics of our society are changing (1). Clearly, patients over the age of 65 represent the most rapidly growing age group. It is estimated that from 2010 to 2020 the population of the United States over the age of 65 will increase by 75%. In addition, during the previous two decades the US population over 85 years of age has grown by 40%. A recent Veterans Administration normative aging study has highlighted the importance of asthma in the aging population. In its study of 894 subjects with a mean age of 60, 12.6% had evidence of increased bronchial hyperresponsiveness; 11% complained of chronic cough; and 7.7% had persistent wheezing. Interestingly, in this patient group only 1.5% of the patients carried a current diagnosis of asthma, which suggests that there is a problem of under-diagnosis or under-recognition of asthma in the elderly. Asthma in the elderly presents a unique challenge to the clinician. This chapter highlights these challenges with special emphasis on the practical considerations for the primary care physician.

Physiologic Changes Caused by Aging

There are many normal physiologic changes caused by aging that can affect airway function in the elderly (Table 11-1) (2). Normal aging is associated with diminished FVC, FEV$_1$, and closing volumes, which can directly affect airway function. Decreased mucous production and cough mechanisms can lead to impairment in clearance of micro-organisms. Impaired thermo-regulation may result in an exaggerated response of airway tone to environmental temperature changes. Atrophy of diaphragmatic and chest wall musculature may further interfere with the mechanics of breathing. Costochondral junctions, which are important in maintaining the normal

---

Table 11-1   Physiologic and Immunologic Changes in the Elderly Patient

- Diminished FEV_1, FVC
- Decreased mucous production
- Decreased cough mechanisms
- Atrophy of diaphragmatic chest muscles
- Impaired specific antibody response
- Impaired T cell response to growth factors and antigens

---

bellows effects of the lungs, can calcify and become degenerative, further impairing airway mechanics. Bronchial smooth muscle fibers atrophy, which could diminish bronchodilatory reserve. Although not one of these normal physiologic effects of aging results in irreversible bronchial hyperresponsiveness associated with asthma, the normal physiologic mechanisms of aging can result in impaired lung function.

Immunologic responses are impaired with advancing age and may have direct or indirect effects on bronchial asthma. Although total antibody levels are normal, there appears to be impaired specific antibody response to antigen. In addition, there appears to be a greater propensity for autoantibody production with increased incidence of antinuclear antibody, rheumatoid factor, and lymphocytotoxic antibodies in the elderly. Impaired cellular immune responses in the aging are well described. There are decreased T-cell responses to growth factors and to specific antigens. Diminished IL-2 production and IL-2 receptor expression may further impair T-cell responses. Although no one immunologic deficit appears to be responsible for the initiation or perpetuation of asthma in the elderly, it is important to recognize that elderly asthmatics may have altered responses to antigens or to medications (e.g., corticosteroids, biological response modifiers) that may further suppress immune responses.

Differential Diagnosis

When considering the diagnosis of asthma in the elderly, the differential diagnosis becomes expanded (Table 11-2) (see Chapter 3) (3). Chronic obstructive pulmonary disease (COPD) is perhaps the most common condition in the differential diagnosis. Although a history of cigarette smoking would certainly suggest this diagnosis, there are some individuals who develop COPD with or without alpha-1 antitrypsin deficiency who lack a history of cigarette smoking. Although COPD patients may have increased nonspecific bronchial hyperresponsiveness, this "asthmatic component" of COPD may need to be treated differently. Pulmonary function studies can be useful in distinguishing asthma from COPD (Table 11-3). Spirometric

Table 11-2   Differential Diagnosis of Asthma in the Elderly Patient

- COPD with emphysema
- Interstitial lung disease
- Bronchiectasis
- Pulmonary embolism
- Gastroesophageal reflux
- Lung carcinoma
- Congestive heart failure (see Case 11-1)
- Rheumatic diseases (rheumatoid arthritis, systemic lupus erythematosus, scleroderma, Sjögren's syndrome)
- Respiratory vasculitic syndromes, Churg-Strauss syndrome, Wegener's granulomatosus

Table 11-3   Differentiating COPD from Asthma in the Elderly

	FEV_1	FEV1/FVC	TLC	DLCO	12%–15% Response to Bronchodilator
Asthma	Decreased	Decreased	Normal	Normal or increased	Usually
Emphysema	Decreased	Decreased	May be increased	Decreased	Rarely

parameters, including FEV_1, FVC, and FEF_{25-75}, are useful in distinguishing chronic airways obstruction from other pulmonary conditions. Measuring the response to a bronchodilator can be extremely helpful in determining the degree of reversibility that is classically associated with asthma.

Although there is no universally accepted criterion for degree of reversibility necessary to establish the presence of reversible obstructive airways disease, a 12% to 15% improvement in FEV_1 expressed as percentage of baseline is frequently utilized for this purpose. It is important to note that the degree of improvement should additionally be at least 200 cc, because many older individuals with severe impairment of lung function may show a dramatic change in percentage, which may represent less than 100 cc and is unlikely to be clinically or physiologically significant. Recent studies have suggested that the criteria for degree of reversibility be downwardly adjusted to 10% because in nonsmoking individuals this degree of reversibility has been found to be greater than 90% sensitive and specific for establishing the diagnosis of asthma. Although the single-breath carbon monoxide diffusing capacity (DLCO) is classically used to distinguish COPD

CASE 11-1   *Elderly man with congestive heart failure mimicking asthma symptoms*

A 76-year-old man presents to the urgent care clinic complaining of a 3-week history of chest congestion and wheezing. He had been in his usual state of health until that time and had been maintained on atenolol and diazide for chronic hypertension and "rapid heartbeat" for the previous 5 years. He denies having any recent episodes of chest pressure. He has no exertional chest pain and no paroxysmal nocturnal dyspnea or orthopnea. There is no obvious change in his weight. He denies having other signs or symptoms of an upper respiratory tract infection and denies fever or purulent sputum production.

His past medical history is otherwise significant for chronic exogenous obesity for the previous 20 years. He has mild diet-controlled diabetes mellitus and hypercholesterolemia. The patient is a retired railroad conductor. He smoked one half to one pack of cigarettes per day for 20 years but has had no cigarette consumption for 20 years. Family history is significant for his having no obviously atopic family members. Environmental history is significant for his living in a high-rise apartment provided with electric heat and his having no animals.

Physical examination reveals the presence of dry mucous membranes of the oropharynx. Examination of the lungs reveals the presence of bilateral end expiratory wheezing without rales. Examination of the heart reveals no obvious signs of cardiac enlargement. There is no S3, S4, or murmurs appreciated. There is 1+ pitting edema of the ankles bilaterallly.

At the time of his presentation he is given a prescription for prn albuterol and fluticasone 110 µg 2 puffs twice daily. He is asked to return to his primary care physician in 2 weeks. At that time there is no change in his symptoms despite the medications. His physical examination is unchanged. A chest x-ray reveals the presence of new cardiomegaly with cephalization of flow. The patient is in mild congestive heart failure for which he is treated with a diuretic. He returns to his primary care physician's office 1 week later, at which time his symptoms of wheezing and chest congestion have entirely abated. He has discontinued his fluticasone and albuterol. In his primary care physician's office spirometry is entirely normal, and he is scheduled for cardiac evaluation, including an exercise thallium test and echocardiogram.

Discussion

Here is a classic demonstration of the adage that "all that wheezes is not asthma." This case is an example of what some refer to as "cardiac asthma," in which the presence of wheezing had suggested to previous examiners that the patient was suffering from asthma when indeed the diagnosis was congestive heart failure.

---

from asthma, it should be noted that the DLCO in and of itself is not entirely diagnostic of COPD. It should be pointed out that some patients with asthma may in fact have elevated DLCOs. When the elevated DLCO associated with asthma is combined with a diminution in the pulmonary capillary vasculature associated with emphysema, patients may have falsely normal DLCOs. Because many elderly asthmatics have smoked in the past, it is important to recognize that COPD and asthma may coexist in many of these patients.

Older individuals may have other underlying parenchymal lung disease such as interstitial lung disease, bronchiectasis, or obliterative bronchiolitis. A diagnosis of interstitial lung disease is usually based on a clinical assessment, which includes history, physical exam, physiologic testing, and imaging studies. Classically, patients with interstitial lung disease describe symptoms of exertional dyspnea and only rarely describe wheezing. Physical examination in a patient with interstitial lung disease classically reveals changes of inspiratory rales that are heard best at the lung bases, which have been referred to as having a "Velcro" characteristic. Chest x-ray or high-resolution computed tomography (CT) scan may reveal the presence of interstitial infiltrates. Spirometric parameters classically reveal restrictive rather than obstructive changes with a normal FEV_1/FVC ratio and reduced lung volumes. Bronchiectasis may be difficult to distinguish from underlying asthma because patients with bronchiectasis may present with cough, shortness of breath, and wheezing. There are no classic physical examination abnormalities that are specific for this condition. Physical examination may reveal the presence of a prolonged expiratory phase and audible wheezing. Chest x-ray or high-resolution CT scanning classically reveals the "tram track" changes indicating the presence of expanded airways.

Pulmonary embolus is more commonly seen in the elderly and should always be considered in the differential diagnosis of a breathless patient. Patients may present with shortness of breath, wheezing episodes, and hypoxia that may masquerade as asthma. Obesity, bed rest, recent surgery, congestive heart failure, cancer, and estrogen treatment all are associated with pulmonary embolism. Furthermore, hypercoagulable states with or without associated malignancy may predispose some elderly individuals to pulmonary embolism. Nevertheless, patients with pulmonary embolism usually have abrupt onset of symptoms and can present with prominent pleuritic chest pain. Their symptoms characteristically do not improve with bronchodilator treatment.

The prevalence of gastroesophageal reflux in the elderly has been estimated to be as high as 20%. The major proposed mechanisms of reflux-induced asthma include 1) the direct microaspiration of gastric contents into the bronchial tree with resultant bronchial spasm, and 2) the reflex bronchoconstriction caused by stimulation of vagal esophageal receptors. Both mechanisms may be involved in asthma in the elderly.

Gastroesophageal reflux may be the primary cause of cough and chest tightness or may be responsible for aggravating underlying asthma. In some cases, severe gastroesophageal reflux can lead to bronchiectasis. Medical therapy with H_2-antagonists or proton-pump inhibitors may be required in high doses for prolonged duration to affect the clinical outcome of asthma in elderly patients with associated gastroesophageal reflux.

Because the incidence of malignancy increases in the elderly, lung cancer must always be included in new-onset or worsening shortness of breath in the elderly. In older adults, bronchogenic carcinoma may present with wheezing and shortness of breath. Whereas shortness of breath may be caused by airway luminal narrowing or ventilation perfusion mismatch, the wheezing heard on examination in patients with lung cancer is usually localized.

Recently the Churg-Strauss syndrome has been recognized as an important diagnostic consideration. Although no cause-and-effect relationship has been established between the use of leukotriene modifiers and Churg-Strauss syndrome, the availability of these and other asthma controller agents (e.g., salmeterol) has allowed clinicians to taper corticosteroids only to unmask an underlying systemic vasculitis. This unique syndrome appears to occur only in patients with underlying asthma and is associated with pulmonary infiltrates, hypereosinophilia, cutaneous leukocytoclastic vasculitis, and/or necrotizing vasculitis of peripheral nerves and the gastrointestinal and cardiovascular systems. The availability of high-resolution CT scanning of the lung has afforded the clinician the opportunity to distinguish this syndrome as well as other conditions from asthma in many cases. It is important to stress that individuals with chronic persistent asthma without other lung diseases may have fibrotic changes on high-resolution CT scanning.

Sometimes it is quite difficult to differentiate primary asthma from "cardiac asthma." For almost two centuries, clinicians have recognized that patients with organic heart disease resulting in elevated left ventricular end diastolic pressures and pulmonary congestion may present with wheezing (4). It is important to stress that the wheezing associated with congestive heart failure may be somewhat improved after administration of a bronchodilator. Every elderly patient who presents with wheezing should be carefully examined for potential signs of congestive heart failure (see Case 11-1). Particular attention should be directed towards the jugular venous pressure, the presence of an audible third or fourth heart sound, or the presence of peripheral edema. A plain chest film can be extremely helpful in distinguishing an elderly patient's cause of breathlessness, because cardiomegaly and pulmonary vascular congestion would certainly point to heart failure. A two-dimensional echocardiogram may be helpful in determining the cause of congestive heart failure by assessing for potential valvular, ischemic, or cardiomyopathic abnormalities. On rare occasions, right-heart catheterization with measurement of pulmonary pressures and cardiac output may be necessary to distinguish cardiac causes of dyspnea and wheezing from reversible obstructive airways disease.

Rheumatic diseases and rheumatic disease treatment can be an important cause of pulmonary disease that may masquerade as asthma in the elderly. Rheumatoid arthritis is perhaps the most important rheumatic disease in the elderly because it affects approximately 1% of the general population and is a multisystem disease that has prominent extra-articular features. These features may include pleurisy with pleural effusions, interstitial fibrosis, bronchiolitis obliterans with or without organizing pneumonia, pulmonary nodules, and pulmonary vasculitis. All of these extra-articular manifestations of rheumatoid arthritis may present with cough and/or breathlessness. Occasionally, elderly patients may in fact have audible wheezing associated with these conditions. Systemic lupus erythematosus is a multisystem autoimmune disease, which, although it normally affects younger women, may have a late onset in 15% to 20% of patients. It is interesting to note that in those women with late-onset systemic lupus erythematosus there is a higher incidence of interstitial pulmonary disease and associated Sjögren's syndrome. Sjögren's syndrome may in fact be the rheumatic disease with the most prominent pulmonary involvement. Patients with Sjögren's syndrome frequently present with interstitial lung disease, cough, and shortness of breath. Systemic sclerosis or scleroderma is an uncommon multisystem autoimmune disorder, with approximately 25% of cases beginning after age 60. Almost all of these patients have prominent esophageal dysmotility and subsequent gastroesophageal reflux, which can result in an "asthmatic" clinical presentation. The most important of the pulmonary manifestations of scleroderma is the presence of pulmonary hypertension. Patients with scleroderma who present with pulmonary hypertension characteristically present with cough and exertional dyspnea and are associated with a poor prognosis. Finally, it should be noted that, in addition to Churg-Strauss syndrome, systemic vasculitic conditions may affect the lungs, including Wegener's granulomatosus and microscopic polyarteritis with pulmonary hemorrhage.

Multiple anti-rheumatic drugs used in elderly individuals can result in drug-induced lung disease. Nonsteroidal anti-inflammatory drugs (NSAIDs) may result in new-onset asthma or trigger of underlying asthma in the elderly. NSAIDs have also been known to induce pulmonary edema. Administration of gold has resulted in the presence of hypersensitivity pneumonitis. The administration of D-penicillamine has resulted in obliterative bronchiolitis and pulmonary hemorrhage. The use of methotrexate can be associated with an acute pneumonitis, which can occur in 2% to 3% of patients maintained on low-dose therapy.

Clinical Presentation

There may be unique aspects to the clinical presentation of asthma in the elderly. Asthma is frequently underdiagnosed in this population (5). Multiple retrospective and longitudinal studies of individuals presenting with new-onset asthma after the age of 65 have indicated that these patients tend to have more persistent and severe disease than do younger patients presenting with new-onset asthma. It is estimated that approximately one half of elderly patients who present with new-onset asthma experience their initial symptoms during or immediately after a respiratory tract infection. Because many individuals in these studies had a previous history of smoking, there are multiple confounding variables. The presenting FEV_1 in elderly patients with new-onset asthma tends to be less than that in those who present with asthma at a younger age, with mean FEV_1 ranging from 60% to 70%. The response to a bronchodilator also appears to be less than that in younger patients. The underlying severity of asthma in the elderly is highlighted by the fact that these individuals have a high utilization of health services. In one study approximately one quarter of elderly patients had emergency room visits for their asthma and almost one half had a hospitalization.

There have been many observations regarding the association of atopy with asthma in the elderly. It is known that both skin test reactivity and serum IgE levels peak in the third decade of life and markedly decline after age 50. Whereas over 80% of children with asthma will have identifiable allergic triggers to their asthma, there appears to be a much lower association with allergic triggers in asthma in individuals after age 50. However, it should be pointed out that while there is a lower incidence of allergen-induced asthma in the elderly, allergen-induced asthma may continue to be a very significant problem in a substantial proportion of asthmatics (Case 11-2). Interestingly, although the overall prevalence of associated nasal polyposis in asthma is 7%, it may be as high as 15% in older asthmatics. In addition, idiosyncratic reactions to NSAIDs resulting in severe asthma are more common in patients with coexisting asthma and nasal polyposis. This condition is known as the *aspirin* or *Samter's triad* (see Chapter 13). It is also important to note that in most retrospective studies of asthma in the elderly many patients have indicated a previous history of childhood allergies or transient episodes of asthma. This history may identify these individuals as being atopic phenotypes, which leads to mild persistent bronchial hyper-responsiveness throughout life.

CASE 11-2   *Elderly woman with new-onset asthma possibly caused by seasonal and perennial allergen exposure*

A 68-year-old woman presents to her primary care physician with a cough that "won't go away." She states that she had been in her usual state of health until approximately 3 months previously when she noted the insidious onset of a nonproductive cough and intermittent shortness of breath and chest congestion. She denies having had an obvious recent upper respiratory tract infection. She denies fever, purulent sputum production, and hemoptysis. She denies chest pain and audible wheezing. She reports intermittent nocturnal awakening caused by her cough three or four times a week. She also notes a definite increase in her cough after heavy exertion such as carrying groceries or mowing her lawn.

Continued

Her review of systems indicates a 1-year history of increasing ocular "irritation," nasal congestion, and sneezing, but is otherwise unremarkable. Her past medical history is unremarkable. She is maintained on no long-term medications and has no known medication allergy. A retired bookkeeper, 8 months before her presentation she had moved to the Pacific Northwest from Colorado Springs to be close to her grandchildren. She is a lifelong nonsmoker and has used no alcohol or recreational drugs. Her family history is significant in that both of her parents died in their mid-80s of "old age." She has two children, including a son with a history of "ragweed hayfever," which occurred in the fall only when he lived in the Midwest. Environmental history is significant for her having two new puppies, which she acquired after the onset of her symptoms. She lives in a newly constructed townhouse with forced-air gas heat and no basement.

Physical examination reveals the presence of marked bilateral nasal turbinate edema and erythema. Examination of the lungs reveals the presence of bilateral end expiratory wheezing. CBC and chemistry panel are unremarkable. A chest x-ray is normal. Office spirometry reveals the presence of a diminished FEV_1 of 68%, FEV_1/FVC ratio of 72%, and FEF_{25-75} 55% of predicted. FEV_1 normalizes to 85% 20 min after the administration of two inhalations of albuterol.

At the time of her initial presentation, the patient is started on prn albuterol and given a daily oral leukotriene modifier. She returns to her primary care physician office in 2 weeks stating that she is approximately 50% improved.

Discussion

This is a case of new-onset asthma in an elderly patient who presents primarily with cough. Although cough was her primary symptom, she also complained of chest congestion and shortness of breath. She had physiologic evidence of reversible obstructive airways disease on spirometric testing, and on physical examination had obvious wheezing. Although a definitive diagnosis is in little question here, the underpinnings of her airway obstruction have not been clearly identified. Despite the fact that she is 68 years old, she has moved from an area in which allergen exposure was minimal to an area of the country where seasonal and perennial allergen exposure is quite significant. This is a case in which identification of potential relevant allergens would be quite helpful. For instance, if she were allergic to dust and dogs, appropriate environmental control measures could be undertaken. It would be important to identify whether she was sensitive to outdoor allergens such as grasses or trees so that appropriate avoidance measures could be recommended.

Therapy

Perhaps the greatest challenge to a clinician caring for the elderly asthmatic is selecting appropriate therapy (Table 11-4) (6). Most elderly patients are taking multiple medications. Furthermore, cognitive dysfunction associated with aging may lead to decreased compliance. The presence of decreased

---

Table 11-4   Therapeutic Considerations for the Elderly Asthmatic Patient

- There is less affinity of β_2-agonist for β_2-receptor.

- Inhaled corticosteroids remain the most effective anti-inflammatory controller agents but may be associated with systemic side effects in high doses.

- Salmeterol is a useful addition to inhaled corticosteroids and allows tapering of corticosteroid dose.

- Leukotriene modifiers are safe and effective options for controller therapy as monotherapy for patients with mild asthma or as an add-on to inhaled corticosteroids.

- Patient should avoid drugs and lifestyle changes that exacerbate gastroesophageal reflux.

Table 11-5   Factors Affecting Pharmacotherapy in the Elderly Asthmatic Patient

- Most elderly patients are maintained on multiple medications.

- Diminished muscle mass and increased fat affect drug distribution.

- Impaired renal and liver function may affect drug clearance.

- Patient may have cognitive dysfunction affecting compliance.

- Patient may have limited financial resources.

---

muscle mass, increased fat, and impaired renal and hepatic function all may significantly alter drug metabolism. Furthermore, limited financial resources in many of our elderly patients may affect the use of costly new drugs or biotechnology products (Table 11-5).

Recently, national and international guidelines have been proposed for the treatment of asthma. These guidelines suggest that the therapeutic goals in asthma should be

1. To suppress airway inflammation with anti-inflammatory drugs
2. To relieve the symptoms of bronchospasm and breathlessness with bronchodilators
3. To maintain normal and near-normal lung function and activity levels on a daily basis
4. To prevent acute exacerbations of asthma during day and night
5. To avoid significant adverse effects from asthma medications

To adequately treat the elderly asthmatic, it is likely that a "controlling" anti-inflammatory agent will be required, because most elderly patients with asthma have chronic persistent disease as opposed to intermittent asthma.

Inhaled corticosteroids remain the most effective anti-inflammatory agents in the treatment of chronic persistent asthma (see Chapter 6). The anti-inflammatory effects of corticosteroids have been well described and are mediated through their effect on gene expression in the nucleus after binding to a specific receptor in the cytoplasm. Corticosteroids may down-regulate the synthesis of several cytokines and adhesion molecules resulting in an anti-inflammatory effect. Furthermore, up-regulation of gene expression of lipocortins and beta-adrenergic receptors that can further benefit an asthmatic person have been described. Although inhaled corticosteroids have the greatest potential therapeutic benefit in asthma, there are a number of concerns that elderly asthmatics may have, which may limit the use of these agents.

For inhaled corticosteroids to be optimally used, patient adherence to regular dosing regimens and sometimes difficult inhalation techniques must be achieved. Unfortunately, many elderly individuals avoid the use of preventive medications that have no immediate effect because of concerns of high cost or toxicity. The use of systemic corticosteroids in the elderly can result in multiple systemic effects; the effects of systemic corticosteroids on bone metabolism, glucose tolerance, cataract formation, and gonadal function are well known to most treating physicians. Because of this potential, every effort should be made to minimize or eliminate the need for oral corticosteroids in the elderly. It is recommended that clinicians focus on minimizing the bioavailability of inhaled corticosteroids in the elderly because these adverse effects need to be minimized. The use of high-potency, low-systemic bioavailability agents (e.g., budesonide, fluticasone, mometazone) should be encouraged in the elderly patient when high-dose inhaled corticosteroid therapy becomes necessary. The availability of add-on agents (e.g., long-acting B_2-agonists, leukotriene modifiers) may allow the tapering of inhaled corticosteroids to the lowest effective dose.

Particular attention should be directed at the potential effects of inhaled glucocorticoids on bone metabolism in the elderly. Because osteoporosis can be associated with devastating complications, clinicians must attempt to avoid systemic corticosteroids or inhaled corticosteroids with high systemic bioavailability. Many recent studies have noted the association of high-dose inhaled corticosteroids with a reduction in serum osteocalcin, a marker of bone formation. The reduction in serum osteocalcin can occur rapidly, and levels return to normal within a week of corticosteroid discontinuation. Although the osteocalcin response to inhaled corticosteroids is much less than that seen with systemic corticosteroids, every effort should be made to diminish any potential effect on bone metabolism in the elderly. Because post-menopausal women have the highest incidence of osteoporosis, particular attention should be directed towards this potential complication in that group. Patients with underlying osteoporosis or who are at high risk for osteoporosis and require the use of systemic or high-dose inhaled corticosteroids should be carefully monitored for the development of drug-induced abnormalities in bone metabolism. In patients in whom systemic corticosteroids or high-dose inhaled corticosteroids with a potential systemic bioavailability cannot be avoided, treatment with estrogen or other anti-osteoporotic agents must be considered.

The availability of leukotriene modifiers during the past decade has allowed clinicians an alternative to inhaled corticosteroids in those patients who require anti-inflammatory therapy for their asthma. Although it is generally accepted that leukotriene modifiers have a less potent effect on inflammation, many studies indicate their effectiveness in elderly individuals as first-line therapy for mild asthma and add-on therapy to inhaled corticosteroids in patients with more severe disease without need for dosage adjustment. Because patients can easily comply with these agents, elderly asthmatics may derive particular benefit from improved compliance with a long-term controlling anti-inflammatory form of therapy.

Ipatroprium bromide can be delivered both as a metered dose inhaler and through nebulizer solution without need for age-adjusted dosing changes. Ipatroprium bromide is particularly helpful in those patients who have chronic cough associated with COPD. Because inhaled ipatroprium is generally considered safe, it is a reasonable agent to be considered in the treatment of the elderly asthmatic. Unfortunately, inhaled ipatroprium rarely can take the place of other β_2-agonists in the elderly patient with more severe disease. This agent should not be considered as an alternative to long-term controlling anti-inflammatory therapy.

Particular attention should be directed towards beta-agonist response in the elderly. Many studies have documented diminished response to beta-agonists in this group. There appears to be less tachycardia, less vasodilation, and less improvement in peak expiratory flow rate after administration of $beta_2$-agonists in the elderly. Physiologically, there is normal density of the $beta_2$-receptor on cell surfaces, but there appears to be less affinity of the receptor for the agonist. It is unclear whether this represents an effect of the aging process or the effect of previous chronic long-term beta-agonist therapy.

Although theophylline is used much less commonly in asthma therapy, there appears to be a resurgence of its use in some centers. It should be pointed out that even with theophylline levels well within the narrow targeted therapeutic range, signs of theophylline toxicity such as tachycardia, tremulousness, and insomnia may limit its use in the elderly.

Because gastroesophageal reflux is so common in the elderly and its effect on asthma so profound, it should be stressed that many drugs may directly diminish lower esophageal sphincter tone, thus potentially worsening gastroesophageal reflux and asthma (see Chapter 14). These drugs include commonly used agents such as calcium-channel blockers and theophylline, benzodiazepines, nicotine, estrogen, and progesterone. Less commonly used medications such as systemic $beta_2$-agonists, anticholinergics, and alpha-adrenergic agents may also adversely affect gastroesophageal reflux by diminishing lower esophageal sphincter tones. These drugs should be used with great caution in the elderly asthmatic. Lifestyle changes in elderly patients with asthma and suspected gastroesophageal reflux should be aggressively promoted. These changes should include abstinence of alcohol and tobacco. Patients should be instructed to decrease their meal size and to refrain from eating meals more than 3 hr before recumbency. Decreased fat and caffeine intake may further improve gastroesophageal reflux.

Charles Reed at the Mayo Clinic points out that many elderly asthmatics may have irreversible airways obstruction (7). He reviewed 242 patients with asthma over the age of 65 and found that there was no correlation with the degree of physiologic impairment as measured by FEV_1 in the duration of asthma. He was able to identify severe asthmatics with lifelong asthma who have normal FEV_1 and conversely identified patients with late-onset asthma of only several months' duration with severe impairment. Importantly, in this group, patients with positive skin prick testing to inhaled allergens such as pollen, dust mites, and animal danders are more likely to have reversibility on pulmonary function testing with $beta_2$-agonists. This observation highlights the importance of recognizing potential inhaled allergen triggers not only in the younger asthmatic but in the elderly asthmatic as well. Reed further hypothesized that irreversible airway obstruction can occur in adults not only on the basis of emphysema associated with smoking but also because of the effects of chronic inflammation on airways remodeling, bronchiectasis, and post-infectious fibrosis. It is important to note that in this series inhaled corticosteroids did not always prevent decreases in airway function, possibly because of the inability of metered-dose inhalers to deposit drugs in the peripheral airways. As more potent inhaled corticosteroids and better delivery systems become available, it will be important to analyze these outcomes in the future.

Summary

The elderly patient population will represent an increasing challenge in the near future. The physiologic changes that occur in normal aging may change the clinical presentation of asthma. The differential diagnoses of asthma in the elderly include many common conditions that may have been otherwise clinically silent, such as COPD, gastroesophageal reflux, and heart failure. Although asthma in the elderly appears to be less allergic in nature than asthma that presents earlier in life, many elderly patients with asthma have significant allergic triggers. The therapy of asthma in the elderly will continue to present significant challenges to the clinician. Not only must we be aware of the potential side effects of primary asthma therapy but potential drug interactions associated with polypharmacy in the elderly may also be quite significant. Although recognizing and treating asthma in the elderly presents many challenges, the tools to go forward and meet these challenges as they emerge are available.

■ ■ ■

Key Points

- Physiologic changes that occur with aging affect airway function in the elderly. These changes include diminished FVC, FEV_1, and closing volumes.

- The differential diagnosis of asthma in the elderly is extensive and includes chronic obstructive pulmonary disease, underlying parenchymal lung disease, pulmonary embolism, gastroesophageal reflux disease, lung carcinoma, congestive heart failure, rheumatic disease, and respiratory vasculitic syndromes.

- Pulmonary function studies can be useful in distinguishing asthma from COPD, the most common condition in the differential diagnosis. An improvement in FEV_1 of 12% to 15% expressed as a percentage of baseline is frequently used.

- Failure of symptoms to improve with bronchodilator treatment helps distinguish pulmonary embolism from asthma.

- In all elderly patients with asthma who experience wheezing, signs of congestive heart failure should be sought. Use of a plain chest film may be helpful in identifying heart failure as the cause of breathlessness.

- In elderly patients with new-onset asthma, the presenting FEV_1 is often less than that in younger patients, and the response to bronchodilator treatment is not as good.

- Because many elderly patients take multiple medications, often have less compliance with drug regimens, and are more susceptible to adverse effects of asthma therapy, great care should be exercised in formulating an appropriate treatment plan.

■ ■ ■

REFERENCES

1. **Montanaro A.** Allergic disease in an aging population. Immunol Allergy Clin N Am. 1997;7:513–20.
2. **Gyetko MR, Toews GB.** Immunology of the aging lung. Clin Chest Med. 1993;14:379–91.
3. **Osborne ML.** Differential diagnosis of bronchial asthma in the elderly. Immunol Allergy Clin N Am. 1997;17:557.
4. **Vossler MR, Kron J.** Impact of asthma therapy on cardiovascular disorders in the elderly. Immunol Allergy Clin N Am. 1997;17:627–44.

5. **Enright PL, McClelland RL, Newman AB, et al.** Underdiagnosis and undertreatment of asthma in the elderly. Cardiovascular Health Study Research Group. Chest. 1999;116:603–13.

6. **Anderson CJ, Bardana EJ.** Asthma in the elderly: interactions to be wary of [Abstract]. J Respir Dis. 1995;16:965–76.

7. **Reed CE.** The natural history of asthma in adults: the problem of irreversibility. J Allergy Clin Immunol. 1999;103:539–47.

12

Occupational Asthma

Emil J. Bardana, Jr., MD

Occupational asthma is by far the most common work-related respiratory disorder in the industrialized world (1). After the skin, the respiratory tract is the most commonly affected organ system in the workplace. It is the final common pathway for all inhaled dusts, gases, fumes, and vapors encountered, and the continuing proliferation of industrial chemicals and polymers makes it impossible even for experienced clinicians to remain abreast of their number or their potential involvement in a variety of irritational or hypersensitivity disorders. These industrial inhalants can induce a spectrum of symptoms starting with simple annoyance when dealing with nonirritating but disagreeable odors, to definite irritational symptoms of the upper and lower respiratory mucosa when modest concentrations of soluble inhalants with irritating properties are encountered. At the other end of the spectrum, there are corrosive agents capable of causing skin burns, ocular damage, and acute inflammatory changes of the nasopharynx, larynx, and bronchi because of their inherent corrosive properties. Finally, there are industrial agents capable of sensitizing a susceptible group of workers (2).

More than 250 chemicals and organic dusts have been implicated as potential causes of new-onset (*de novo*) occupational asthma, rhinitis, and other hypersensitivity lung disorders. In addition to these industrial agents, a variety of commonly encountered environmental pollutants may also contribute to the development of respiratory ill health in workers. These include indoor and outdoor pollutants, climatic factors, tobacco smoke, and ambient allergens. All of these industrial agents and environmental pollutants must be taken into account by the physician when evaluating patients with suspected occupational asthma (2). Work-related respiratory disease can cause significant morbidity as well as time lost from work. For these reasons, accurate and timely diagnosis is highly desirable. This overview focuses on the classification, pathogenesis, and diagnosis of occupational asthma.

Definition

Occupational asthma is an increasingly common condition that is character-ized by variable airway obstruction and bronchial hyper-responsiveness. It is caused by acute and chronic bronchial inflammation, which has its origin in the inhalation of ambient dusts, vapors, gases, or fumes that are manu-factured or used by the worker or incidentally present at the workplace. A characteristic feature of all chronic symptomatic asthma is the excessive ir-ritability of the airways to a wide variety of environmental stimuli. The airway hyperreactivity is variable and generally correlates with changes in the severity of asthma. It is also evident that many cases of work-related asthma occur in association with chronic bronchitis and varying degrees of irreversible obstructive airway disease (e.g., emphysema).

New-onset or *de novo* occupational asthma can develop as a result of two fundamentally different pathogenetic pathways (2). The more common pathway involves sensitization to a workplace allergen (i.e., immunologic occupational asthma). The second, less common, mechanism is via an ex-posure to a corrosive agent resulting in acute inflammatory bronchospasm (i.e., nonimmunologic occupational asthma). Occupational asthma may also develop in an individual with pre-existing asthma. Such an individual may experience a transient, irritational expression of pre-existing asthma secondary to workplace irritants. This is the most common presentation to the general internist. As well, a patient with pre-existent asthma may have a significant encounter with a truly corrosive agent that permanently worsens the pre-existing condition. Alternatively, an atopic patient with pre-existing asthma may develop a unique sensitization to a workplace allergen.

When evaluating any patient for work-related asthma, it is critical to con-sider the diagnosis in the context of the lifelong medical history. Any pre-exist-ing lung condition should be considered a potential contributor to the suspected work-related asthma. Disorders that are sometimes overlooked include bullous disease of the lungs, bronchiectasis, emphysema, chronic bronchitis, sarcoido-sis, and collagen-vascular disorders. In addition, several upper respiratory dis-orders may accentuate or contribute to asthmatic symptoms. The latter include conditions such as allergic rhinoconjunctivitis, nasal polyposis associated with aspirin-sensitivity syndrome, and chronic or recurrent pyogenic sinusitis.

Epidemiology

Reliable data on the prevalence of occupational asthma have been difficult to determine. The obstacles that make this difficult include

1. The variability of definitions for work-related asthma
2. The retrospective approach to almost all previous clinical research that characterizes much of the available information

3. Geographic differences in the nature of the industries

4. Industrial hygiene practices and likely exposures

5. Availability of current statistics reflecting modern industrial hygiene standards

6. The variability of state workers' compensation statutes and reporting practices.

There are no long-term controlled, prospective, perspective studies of occupational asthma. In addition, nearly all epidemiologic studies have relied upon subjective data in identifying asthma. Hence, in most cohorts studied, it is not possible to ascertain whether minimally symptomatic, undiagnosed, nonoccupational asthma was present before any putative exposure.

With these caveats in mind, it has been estimated that 15 million people in the United States have bronchial asthma. The prevalence of occupational asthma is said to range from 2% to 6% of the asthmatic population. Consistent with this estimate, a recent large population-based study of occupational asthma estimated that between 5% and 10% of cases of asthma among young adults in European and other industrialized countries were secondary to occupational exposures (3). Unfortunately, this study did not distinguish between *de novo* occupational asthma and pre-existing asthma that was exacerbated because of an occupational exposure.

There has been a tendency to derive prevalence information by evaluating specific industries in different regions of the world. However, industry-specific information cannot be reliably extrapolated to comparable industries worldwide. For example, reports of work-related asthma affecting 7% to 9% of unselected bakers is more consistent with European family-run bakeries than with the large production facilities of North America. Most industry-specific prevalence rates represent older studies under primitive work conditions that are no longer applicable in the majority of well-run modern manufacturing facilities with established safety programs.

Many investigators believe that the 5% prevalence figure represents an underestimation. They argue that a significant number of workers become ill with occupational asthma and leave the industry without reporting their illness, creating a resistant "survivor population." As well, they argue that other affected workers remain at their job and fail to report their disease for fear of losing their job and/or their seniority. An additional group of workers is said to be misdiagnosed. These observations must be counterbalanced by equally cogent considerations that in a medical system where workers are highly protected by state workers' compensation statutes, it is highly unlikely that a worker would remain silent in the face of significant work-related disease. Additionally, in an increasingly competitive system in which medical insurance may be lacking or inadequate, there is a tendency to invoke the possibility of occupational illness as a strategy to ensure reimbursement from the workers' compensation system. Finally, there are those workers who have abused the system for personal secondary gain.

Predisposing Factors

The development of occupational asthma may be influenced by a variety of genetic, industrial, climatic, social, and medical factors (Table 12-1).

Workplace Factors

The issues that may impact worker injury or illness relate to the extent and nature of possible chemical exposures as well as both the employer's and employee's attitude toward safety programs (e.g., availability of material safety data sheets (MSDS), adequate protective equipment, adherence to safety procedures, implementation of effective industrial hygiene measures).

Climatic Conditions

A variety of meteorological conditions have been implicated in the modification of worker response to inhaled antigens. Several asthma epidemics in Barcelona, Spain between 1981 and 1987 were attributed to large amounts of soybean dust released into the ambient atmosphere with subsequent deposition onto nearby roadways on days when wind velocity was low. In addition, certain outdoor pollutants have been found to facilitate the development of sensitization to prevailing allergens. This has been shown with oxides of nitrogen as well as diesel exhaust particles. Ozone is said to potentiate the response to inhaled allergen in sensitized subjects.

**Table 12-1   Predisposing Factors Influencing the Development of
De Novo Occupational Asthma**

- Workplace factors
  —Chemical sources and their ambient
    concentrations
  —Industrial hygiene practices
  —Safety policy adherence
- Climatic variables
  —High levels of oxidizing pollutants
  —Temperature inversions
  —Wind conditions
  —Seasonal allergens
- Genetic features
  —Allelic polymorphisms associated
    with atopic state

- Tobacco and recreational drug use
- Respiratory infections
  —Viral infections that may
    precipitate asthma
  —*Mycoplasma* or *Chlamydia*
    infections
  —Pyogenic sinus infections
- Bronchial hyperreactivity
- Miscellaneous factors
  —Aspirin-sensitivity syndrome
  —Gastroesophageal reflux
  —Pharmaceutical agents

Genetics

A personal or family history of atopic disease (e.g., hayfever, asthma, atopic eczema) may be helpful in evaluating occupational asthma because atopic subjects develop work-related asthma more readily than do nonatopic individuals exposed to the same agents. This is particularly true with respect to industries in which high-molecular-weight (HMW) agents are involved (e.g., animal handlers, grain and flour handlers, seafood processors) (Table 12-2). There is convincing evidence that atopy plays a role in the development of bronchial asthma, bronchial hyperresponsiveness, and other allergic disorders (4). It is therefore logical that atopic subjects are more likely to develop occupational asthma when exposed to high- and selected low-molecular-weight agents. Genetic research related to atopic linkages has demonstrated allelic polymorphisms associated with genes encoding the β-subunit of the high-affinity IgE receptor, regulatory cytokines, the β_2-receptor, and the IL-4 α-receptor. Furthermore, there is now mounting evidence that asthma and sensitization to low-molecular-weight chemicals encountered at work are influenced by HLA polymorphisms (5).

Tobacco and Recreational Drug Use

There are approximately 50 million Americans who smoke tobacco. They place not only themselves at risk but also those who are passively exposed. Several groups of investigators have incriminated cigarette smoking as both a predisposing and an aggravating factor in the development of occupational

Table 12-2   Selected Asthmogenic Agents Categorized by Molecular Weight

High-Molecular-Weight Allergens	Low-Molecular-Weight Immunogens
• Insect parts	• Platinum salts
• Mammalian proteins	• Penicillins
• Avian proteins	• Cephalosporins
• Fish-derived allergens	• Sulfonamides
• Fungal allergens	• Nickel
• Grain dust	• Vanadium
• Green coffee bean dust	• Diisocyanates
• Castor bean dust	• Epoxy amine compounds
• Latex allergens	• Colophony
• Vegetable grains	• Western red cedar (plicatic acid)
• Psyllium	• Reactive azo dyes
• Enzymes	

asthma. Smoking is definitely linked to bronchial inflammation with the development of obstructive pulmonary disease. There is a clear relationship between smoking and the presence of bronchial hyperreactivity. Smoking has also been associated with a higher incidence of respiratory infections.

In addition to tobacco abuse, it has been said that regular marijuana smoking is practiced by some 20 million Americans. Sometimes this is in addition to regular tobacco use, and sometimes it is the only smoking practiced. A number of studies have shown that consumption of a few marijuana cigarettes has the potential to cause the same degree of epithelial damage as a larger number of tobacco cigarettes. The latter relates to the usual deep inhalation associated with marijuana smoking and the number of particles retained in the lung. The current widespread smoking of the alkaloidal form of cocaine (crack) has been associated with a variety of severe pulmonary sequelae, including allergic alveolitis, obliterative bronchiolitis, bronchial asthma, and pulmonary edema.

Respiratory Infections

Viral respiratory infections are frequently the initial precipitating event in the onset of bronchial asthma (6). Bronchial hyperreactivity has been associated with viral respiratory infections in both atopic and nonatopic individuals. There are a variety of diverse mechanisms proposed for the association between viral infections and bronchial asthma. These include epithelial injury, development of viral-specific IgE, leukocyte-dependent inflammation, and enhanced mediator release. In general, bacterial infections of the lung are not associated with exacerbations of asthma. However, several exceptions have been noted, including infections with *Mycoplasma pneumoniae* and *Chlamydia pneumoniae*. Pyogenic infections of the paranasal sinuses are also frequently associated with a deterioration of underlying asthma (see Chapter 9).

Nonspecific Bronchial Hyperreactivity

Bronchial hyperreactivity is considered a major characteristic of active bronchial asthma. It is defined as an exaggerated airway narrowing in response to a wide variety of stimuli. It is almost universally present in symptomatic, untreated patients with asthma. Its presence correlates with bronchoalveolar inflammatory cell infiltrate, particularly eosinophils and metachromatic cells. Airway inflammation may be enhanced by a variety of asthmogenic agents including protein allergens, workplace chemical sensitizers, viral agents, ozone, and a variety of other irritating pollutants.

Miscellaneous Factors

A number of unrelated miscellaneous factors may also be associated with the precipitation or aggravation of pre-existent asthma and should be considered in the evaluation of any patient with possible work-related asthma. Diagnostic considerations that should be excluded include aspirin-induced asthma, gastroesophageal reflux, and a variety of pharmaceutical agents that are known to have an adverse effect on the course of asthma. Prime examples are beta-adrenergic blocking agents and angiotensin-converting enzyme inhibitors. These issues are addressed in other chapters.

Clinical and Pathogenic Features

The development of work-related asthma in response to any particular industrial agent is entirely dependent on the type, source, and concentration of the industrial exposure, work conditions, industrial hygiene factors, climatic influences, and the individual characteristics of the host response. This concept partially explains why acute high-level exposures to selected industrial irritants such as toluene diisocyanate might provoke acute inflammatory bronchoconstriction in one instance, whereas chronic low-level exposures to the same agent may induce an immunologic or pharmacologic work-related disorder in another instance (Fig. 12-1). For discussion purposes in this overview, occupational asthma is divided into two broad groups: immunologic and nonimmunologic. Immunologic can be further divided into classic IgE-mediated and polyimmunologic variants. The nonimmunologic variety includes acute inflammatory bronchospasm, also referred to as reactive airways dysfunction syndrome (RADS), reflex bronchoconstriction, and pharmacologic bronchoconstriction.

New-Onset Immunologic Asthma

A large number of industrial agents are capable of inducing an immunologic response resulting in clinical sensitization. Most commonly, the antigens involved are high-molecular-weight allergens, predominantly proteins derived from animals, plants, foods, and enzymes (see Table 12-2) (2). The work exposure usually involves contact with soluble proteins, glycoproteins, or other peptide-containing moieties, which in a predisposed individual causes production of specific IgE antibody. There are also many low-molecular-weight sensitizers that act as haptens and cross-link with plasma proteins to induce typical IgE-mediated responses.

The acid anhydrides and the diisocyanates represent a group of chemicals capable of inducing a variety of respiratory syndromes involving both IgG- and IgE-specific antibody as well as cellular immune mechanisms. These highly reactive, low-molecular-weight compounds have received a great deal of attention from a variety of investigators and serve as models for the diversity of clinical and immunopathologic syndromes that can arise with similar exposures (e.g., polyimmunologic mechanisms) (see Fig.12-1). Despite the advances that have been achieved in the area of

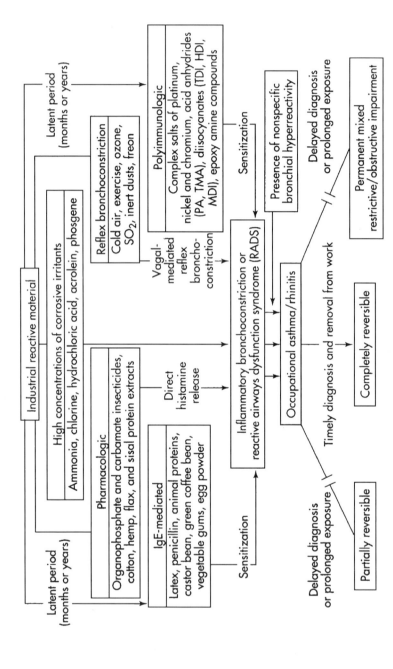

Figure 12-1 Schematic conceptualization of several pathogenetic mechanisms of occupationally induced airway obstruction. (Data from Bardana EJ. Occupational asthma and related respiratory disorders. Dis Mon. 1995;61:141–200.)

occupational asthma, there remain a number of industrial agents associated with occupational asthma for which the pathogenesis remains poorly understood. The two largest groups of chemicals in this category include certain wood dusts and a variety of copolymerizing compounds or hardening agents used in the manufacture of resins or plastics (see Table 12-2) (Case 12-1).

The clinical presentation of the patient with IgE-mediated work-related asthma parallels the symptoms of most patients with classic allergic disorders. Many patients report preceding or concomitant upper airway and ocular symptoms of sneezing, nasal discharge, tearing, and nasal obstruction. There usually is a latent period of months or years before lower respiratory symptoms develop. Patients report work-related airflow obstruction characterized by chest tightness, cough, and dyspnea, which may intensify during the work week. Onset of symptoms with work exposures may be immediate, delayed, or biphasic (dual), consistent with the early- and late-phase allergic responses.

CASE 12-1 *Plywood mill worker with new-onset immunologic asthma caused by western red cedar dust*

A 49-year-old plywood mill worker with an established history of mild seasonal allergic rhinitis presents to his primary care physician with complaints of persistent rhinoconjunctivitis 6 months after starting work as a bandsaw operator of cedar shakes. Over the previous several weeks he further noticed chest tightness, nonproductive cough, and breathlessness, especially at his work. The patient has never smoked, and there have been no changes in his home environment for the previous decade. He denies any evidence of upper respiratory infection, sinusitis, or bronchitis.

Physical examination reveals a body temperature of 37°C, blood pressure 138/72, pulse 78, and respiratory rate of 18/min. The conjunctiva appears reddened, and there is boggy edema of both inferior turbinates. Auscultation of the lungs reveals bilateral diffuse wheezing. Cardiac sounds are normal.

Spirometry shows an FEV_1 of 72% of predicted with an FEV_1/FVC ratio of 64%. Following nebulized bronchodilator the FEV_1 improves to 96% of predicted with a ratio of 78%. A diagnosis of possible occupational asthma is considered.

The patient is advised to remain home from work for 1 week, and he is treated aggressively with bronchodilators. He is asked to discontinue medications 24 hr before a follow-up visit the morning of his return to work, the purpose of which is to avoid masking the possible effects of the anticipated work provocation. Repeat spirometry is normal. Upon return to work, symptoms redevelop over the course of his day, and upon completion of his shift spirometry reveals a 26% decrease in FEV_1. A diagnosis of western red cedar asthma is established, and the patient is transferred to another plywood mill where western red cedar is not being used.

New-Onset Nonimmunologic Asthma

Nonallergic industrial asthma usually results from a high-level exposure to a corrosive irritant in the workplace (Case 12-2). For several thousand years, toxic gases have been recognized as potentially irritating, and even lethal, to the respiratory tract (Table 12-3). The effects of any acute exposure depend on the physiochemical properties of the dust, gas, fume, or vapor involved, as well as specific host factors (Fig. 12-2). Acute injury can be inflicted by avariety of irritant gases and vapors, depending on their water solubility.

CASE 12-2   *Factory worker with new-onset nonimmunologic asthma caused by brief but intense exposure to chlorine gas*

A 32-year-old pulp and paper worker is in an excellent state of health until the day he is exposed to a cloud of chlorine gas after an accidental rupture of a storage tank at the bleach end of a paper and pulp plant. He has no escape mask and is forced to run through the highly irritating gas gasping and coughing for air. He is taken to the plant nurse acutely dyspneic and with stinging in both eyes, nasal irritation, and hoarseness. He is immediately transferred by ambulance to a local emergency room.

Examination reveals a temperature of 37.6°C, blood pressure 152/92, pulse 114/min, and respiratory rate of 24/min. Oxygen saturation is 89%. Examination reveals erythematous conjunctiva, congested and erythematous nasal passages, and an injected posterior pharynx. Auscultation of the chest reveals decreased breath sounds with diffuse high-pitched wheezing. Cardiac sounds are normal.

Pulmonary function studies show an FEV_1 of 78% of predicted, which improves to 93% of predicted after bronchodilators. Chest x-ray is normal.

The patient responds to nebulized bronchodilator and is discharged with a 3-week tapered course of corticosteroids as well as inhaled corticosteroids. A follow-up visit 2 months later reveals the patient to be minimally symptomatic, with a normal examination and spirometry. Methacholine challenge test is positive at a concentration of 5 mg/mL. A follow-up visit 3 months later reveals no symptoms, a normal examination, normal spirometry, and a negative methacholine challenge test. All medication has been discontinued with no recurrence of symptoms.

Table 12-3   Industrial Agents Most Often Incriminated in Causation of Reactive Airways Dysfunction Syndrome

• Toluene diisocyanate	• Phosphoric acid
• Chlorine	• Hydrochloric acid
• Phosgene	• Hydrogen sulfide
• Sulfuric acid	• Anhydrous ammonia
• Smoke inhalation	

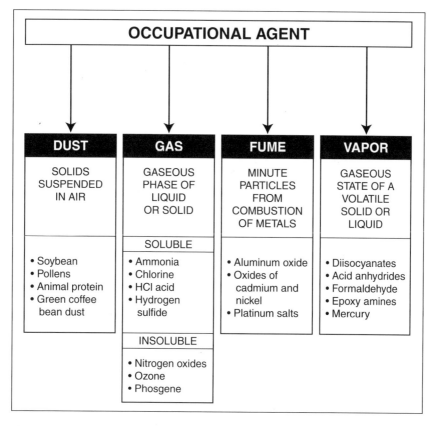

Figure 12-2   Schematic diagram defining the basic physical forms of inhaled work-related substances that determine which part of the lungs will likely be affected. (Data from Bardana EJ. Occupational asthma and related respiratory disorders. Dis Mon. 1995;61:141–200.)

The highly soluble gases (ammonia, chlorine, formaldehyde, etc.) are most likely to cause pharyngeal and laryngeal injury resulting in laryngeal edema. Such exposures are usually associated with facial skin burns, ocular irritation, nasal erythema, and swelling. Most of these soluble gases are absorbed by the mucous membranes of the upper airways. In contrast, the relatively insoluble gases (phosgene, hydrogen sulfide, oxides of nitrogen, etc.) cause little or no upper airway irritation or tissue damage and are much more likely to be associated with intense pulmonary edema, bronchiolitis, and alveolitis after acute high-level exposures. Low-level chronic exposures to certain dusts, gases, and fumes may induce chronic pulmonary conditions such as asbestosis and silicosis.

Historically, the development of new-onset occupational asthma related to a high-level workplace exposure was initially reported in Australia. Four workers developed new-onset asthma after workplace exposure to excessive concentrations of gases and vapors such as hydrogen sulfide and overheated plastics. Clinically its onset was abrupt and not preceded by typical allergic upper airway or ocular complaints. This was initially referred to as *acute inflammatory bronchoconstriction*, but more recently it has been termed *reactive airways dysfunction syndrome* (RADS). RADS is defined as the sudden onset of asthma after a high-level exposure to a corrosive gas, vapor, or fume (see Table 12-3). There exists some controversy related to the criteria necessary to establish this diagnosis.

The clinical presentation of RADS is quite different from that of new-onset immunologic occupational asthma. In RADS, the exposure is characteristically acute, singular, and extreme in nature. In almost all instances, the exposure results from a sudden, unanticipated accident (e.g., a chemical spill or rupture of a container in an area of poor ventilation). There is no latency period such as one finds in typical allergic work-related asthma. Additionally, the exposure is unusual and often lasts only a few minutes. Symptoms of airway obstruction are generally immediate or certainly develop within a few hours of exposure, requiring the afflicted worker to immediately seek emergency care.

The diagnosis of RADS requires the presumption of previous normal pulmonary physiology and absence of bronchial hyper-reactivity. It is also highly dependent on a compatible presentation and the demonstration of persistent, nonspecific, bronchial hyper-responsiveness. Criteria proposed by the American College of Chest Physicians (7) are given in Table 12-4 along with several minor criteria that have been recently proposed (8). The latter

---

Table 12-4   Proposed Criteria for the Diagnosis of Reactive Airways Dysfunction Syndrome

Major Criteria (as proposed by American College of Chest Physicians) (7)
- Absence of previous respiratory complaints
- Onset of symptoms after a single exposure incident
- Exposure to an extremely high concentration of an irritating industrial agent
- Onset of symptoms within 24 hr after exposure, with persistence of symptoms for at least 3 months
- Symptoms simulating asthma
- Presence of airflow obstruction on pulmonary function testing and/or presence of nonspecific bronchial hyperresponsiveness
- All other respiratory disorders excluded

Minor Criteria (8)
- Absence of an atopic state
- Absence of peripheral and pulmonary eosinophilia
- Absence of cigarette smoking for 10 years
- Bronchial hyperreactivity of moderate-to-severe degree (e.g., positive at methacholine concentration ≤ 8 mg/mL)
- Histopathology and/or bronchoalveolar lavage showing minimal lymphocytic inflammation

criteria, if met, strengthen the diagnosis considerably. Satisfaction of at least four of the five minor criteria (including the first three) would exclude the significant confounding factors that inhibit the confident diagnosis of RADS.

The long-term expected outcome for patients with RADS has not been reliably established. Individuals with well-documented RADS may continue to report bronchial irritability symptoms and demonstrate nonspecific bronchial hyperresponsiveness for years after the precipitating event. Recent reports have indicated that if symptoms do not clear within 6 months, they are likely to persist for years. It has also been stated that those who survive the short-term exposure to a corrosive gas, fume, or vapor generally recover completely without significant clinical or physiologic sequelae, regardless of the severity of their initial presentation (7).

In addition to RADS, the most common variant of new-onset nonimmunologic asthma, selected industrial agents may induce bronchospasm by virtue of a direct pharmacologic effect on the respiratory mucosa (see Fig. 12-1). Examples of *pharmacologic bronchoconstriction* are those that can occur with organophosphate and carbamate insecticides. In sufficient doses, these agents inhibit acetylcholinesterase, which potentiates the effect of acetylcholine released from vagal fibers innervating bronchial smooth muscles and promoting bronchoconstriction. There is also some data to suggest that isocyanates can act as pharmacologic inhibitors, reducing the ability of β-adrenergic receptors to produce cyclic AMP levels in sufficient quantities necessary to maintain bronchial tone.

Reflex bronchoconstriction is the third variant of nonallergic occupational asthma. It is distinguished from RADS primarily in the intensity and nature of the inciting exposure. In RADS, the exposure is characteristically acute and extreme, whereas in reflex bronchospasm, the exposure may be sustained and mild to moderate in nature. Certain chemicals and inert gases are thought to have the capacity to cause reflex bronchospasm by disrupting the delicate balance of adrenergic control involved in maintaining bronchial tone. This is thought to be mediated via the irritant receptors in the bronchial wall. It is highly unlikely that this mechanism can induce new-onset (*de novo*) occupational asthma. More likely, it is operative in subjects with pre-existing asthma (i.e., the putative irritant precipitates a transient symptomatic expression of a pre-existing asthmatic condition). A variety of low-level irritants may induce this type of reflex bronchospasm, including ozone, sulfur dioxide, freon, and so on. Permanent residual effects are not generally a feature of this mechanism.

Diagnosis

Differential Diagnosis

In establishing the diagnosis of work-related asthma, the first step must be to establish that asthma truly exists. The second step should be to exclude the possibility that the asthma is of a nonoccupational nature. This is especially true if the worker is atopic and the possibility of subclinical asthma may have been present or simply incorrectly diagnosed for many years. Thirdly, the clinician should exclude other unusual and non-occupational variants of asthma such as allergic bronchopulmonary aspergillosis, aspirin-sensitivity syndrome, Churg-Strauss allergic granulomatosis, and emphysema. Finally, a variety of unrelated pulmonary disorders that can masquerade as asthma must be excluded, including tracheobronchitis, congestive heart failure, vocal cord dysfunction, gastroesophageal reflux disease, and hypersensitivity pneumonitis (see Chapter 3).

History and Physical Examination

The medical history is a critical aspect of the evaluation and should always include a comprehensive review of previous medical records (2). Because of the limited time that may be available, a questionnaire may be used as a tool to amplify the interview process. Anyone who is to be evaluated for the possibility of work-related asthma should be prepared to provide a clear chronological medical history before and after any potentially harmful work exposures. The history should reflect all previous employers and workers' compensation claims and a clear description of the industrial aspects of the workplace. It is also important to acquire a detailed understanding of the protective equipment used by the patient, including facemask, earplugs, goggles, and gloves. The clinician should inquire about the details of any mask worn, how it was fit tested, frequency of cartridge change, presence of prefilters, and so on. Having the worker provide all of the pertinent Material Safety Data Sheets (MSDS) can be extremely helpful (Fig. 12-3).

The physical examination should be carefully carried out to record the presence of ocular, nasal, oropharyngeal, and pulmonary abnormalities. In evaluating any patient with presumptive occupational asthma, the examiner must be completely satisfied that the patient has reversible airflow obstruction (9). Results from a single test have very limited sensitivity and specificity for asthma. Maximal specificity for asthma follows when ventilatory tests are conducted before and after the use of nebulized bronchodilators.

In those instances in which the medical history is compelling yet the reversible airways obstruction is not apparent, an assessment of nonspecific bronchial hyperreactivity can be helpful (i.e., a methacholine challenge test). The diagnostic value of minimal or mild bronchial hyperreactivity must be evaluated cautiously because the presence of bronchial hyperreactivity in the normal population is much higher than previously suspected.

A provisional cause-and-effect relationship with a suspected workplace agent can be developed by serial determination of peak expiratory flow rates during a period of work abstinence and after a return to work (Fig. 12-4) (9). The information gleaned from this exercise should be interpreted with some caution because the maneuver is effort-dependent and can be verified only

<table>
<tr><td colspan="4" align="center">MATERIAL SAFETY DATA SHEET</td></tr>
</table>

MATERIAL SAFETY DATA SHEET			
I PRODUCT IDENTIFICATION			
MANUFACTURER'S NAME	REGULAR TELEPHONE NO. EMERGENCY TELEPHONE NO.		
ADDRESS			
TRADE NAME			
SYNONYMS			
II HAZARDOUS INGREDIENTS			
MATERIAL OR COMPONENT		HAZARD DATA	
III PHYSICAL DATA			
BOILING POINT 760 MM HG		MELTING POINT	
SPECIFIC GRAVITY (H$_2$0=1)		VAPOR PRESSURE	
VAPOR DENSITY (AIR=1)		SOLUBILITY IN H$_2$0 % BY WT	
% VOLATILES BY VOL		EVAPORATION RATE IBUTYL ACETATE II	
APPEARANCE AND ODOR			

Figure 12-3   Format of a Material Safety Data Sheet (MSDS). Daytime and emergency telephone numbers are usually located in the upper right-hand corner of the front page. Peak flow is seen to drop 40% by the fourth day of work. (Data from Bardana EJ. Occupational asthma and related respiratory disorders. Dis Mon. 1995;61:141–200.)

when executed under direct observation using published guidelines. An alternative and more secure approach to the diagnosis is to compare the degree of nonspecific bronchial hyperreactivity after a period of continuous occupational exposure with a point following a 3- to 4-week total abstinence from the suspected agent. Provided there are no significant changes in medication, a change in bronchial reactivity greater than two doubling concentrations (or doses) is considered significant. A third approach is to rely on cross-shift spirometric data (i.e., pre- and post-shift spirometry) over the course of a work week (9).

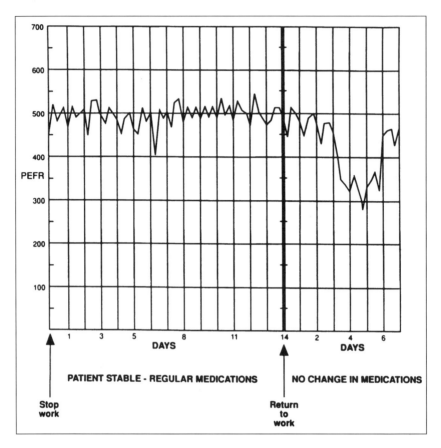

Figure 12-4   Schematic representation of serial peak expiratory flow rates charted during a period of work abstinence and after a return to work. Peak-flow is seen to drop by 40% by the fourth day of work. (Data from Bardana EJ. Occupational asthma and related respiratory disorders. Dis Mon. 1995;61:141–200.)

The absolute gold standard in the diagnosis of allergic occupational asthma is a controlled bronchial challenge with subirritant concentrations of the suspected immunogen. A variety of excellent protocols have been developed for such a study. Because provocation studies pose potential risks to the patient, patients must be appropriately informed and consent must be obtained for the procedure. These studies must be conducted by experienced clinicians, preferably in a hospital setting.

Prevention and Management

The most effective way of preventing occupational asthma is to insulate at-risk workers from potentially hazardous agents. This requires the employer to adopt ideal industrial hygiene measures that will reduce ambient levels of known irritants or immunogens to the lowest possible levels, or to remove them entirely from the industrial process. This can be accomplished by utilization of an approved respirator, by highly effective exhaust ventilation, or by installation of an enclosed automated process such as robotics. Additionally, many employers are installing regular surveillance programs to monitor the respiratory health of employees, including annual spirometric examinations.

The principles of managing symptomatic occupational asthma are the same as those for nonoccupational asthma. Combinations of anti-inflammatory and bronchodilator drugs are advocated (see Chapter 6). It is, however, critical to remember that continued exposure to the offending industrial agent will very likely worsen the condition. The most effective treatment for occupational asthma is removal of the afflicted individual from further exposure as promptly as possible. Experts agree that the single most significant determinant of prognosis is the length of exposure before diagnosis. After removal from further exposure, most patients with occupational asthma experience some improvement in their symptoms. Nevertheless, there are some workers who continue to manifest symptoms and who may require further evaluation to determine the extent of permanent impairment.

■   ■   ■

Key Points

- Occupational asthma is an increasingly common condition caused by acute and chronic bronchial inflammation resulting from inhalation of ambient dust, vapors, gases, or fumes manufactured at the workplace.

- Individuals with or without pre-existing asthma may develop occupational asthma. It may develop as an allergic sensitization to a workplace allergen, as an irritational expression of pre-existing asthma secondary to workplace irritants, or as an acute worsening due to a significant exposure to a corrosive agent in the workplace.

- Occupational asthma can be divided into two groups: immunologic and nonimmunologic asthma.

- The causative antigens of immunologic asthma are high-molecular-weight allergens such as grain dust and proteins from animals and fish. Symptoms occur after a latent period of months to years.

- Nonimmunologic asthma is caused by a brief high-level exposure to a corrosive irritant. Symptoms occur immediately or within a few hours of the exposure. Symptoms may persist for a few months to many years.

■   ■   ■

REFERENCES

1. **Blanc PD, Eisner MD, Israel L, Yelin EH.** The association between ocupation and asthma in general medical practice. Chest. 1999;115:1259–64.
2. **Bardana EJ.** Occupational asthma and related respiratory disorders. Dis Mon. 1995;61:141–200.
3. **Kogevinas M, Anto JM, Sunyer J, et al.** Occupational asthma in Europe and other industrialized areas: a population-based study. Lancet. 1999;353:1750–4.
4. **Holgate ST.** Genetic and environmental interaction in allergy and asthma. J Allergy Clin Immunol. 1999;104:1139–46.
5. **Newman Taylor AJ, Cullman P, Lympany PA, et al.** Interaction of HLA phenotype and exposure intensity in sensitization to complex platinum salts. Am J Respir Crit Care Med. 1999;160:431–8.
6. **Busse WW, Gern JE.** Viruses in asthma. J Allergy Clin Immunol. 1997;100:147–50.
7. **Alberts WM, doPico G.** Reactive airways dysfunction syndrome. Chest. 1996;104: 1618–26.
8. **Bardana EJ.** Reactive airways dysfunction syndrome (RADS): guidelines for diagnosis and treatment and insight into likely prognosis. Ann Allergy Asthma Immunol. 1999;83:583–6.
9. **Tan RA, Spector SL.** Diagnostic testing in occupational asthma. Ann Allergy Asthma Immunol. 1999;83:587–92.

SELECTED READING

Bardana EJ, Montanaro A. Occupational asthma and related disorders. In: Rich RR, et al, eds. Clinical Immunology: Principles and Practice, 2nd ed. St. Louis: Mosby; 2001:57.1–57.14.

Bernstein IL, Chan-Yeung M, Malo JL, Bernstein DI, eds. Asthma in the Workplace, 2nd ed. New York: Marcel Dekker; 1999.

13

Drug-Induced Asthma

Donald D. Stevenson, MD

Very few events in medicine are more distressing to the physician than inducing adverse reactions in patients with prescribed medications. This chapter discusses asthma induced by aspirin, or acetylsalicylic acid (ASA), and other nonsteroidal anti-inflammatory drugs (NSAIDs) and by beta-blocker medications and angiotensin converting enzyme (ACE) inhibitors. There is no relationship between NSAIDs, beta-blockers, and ACE inhibitors; the mechanisms and severity of the various reactions to these drugs are entirely different. Evidence that any of these drugs actually causes asthma has never been shown. These drugs *worsen* ongoing asthma, particularly if the asthma is already out of control. Other topics include the safety of COX-2 inhibitors in all asthmatic patients, including those who are sensitive to ASA/NSAIDs, and the controversial role of ACE inhibitors in the induction of asthma activity.

ASA/NSAID Induced Asthma

ASA/NSAIDs can induce rhinorrhea, laryngospasm, and bronchospasm in some patients with underlying rhinosinusitis and asthma. Various terms have been used to describe the respiratory reactions to NSAIDs: *ASA intolerance, ASA idiosyncrasy, pseudo-allergic respiratory reactions, ASA induced asthma,* and *ASA sensitivity.*

ASA and the other NSAIDs, all of which inhibit cyclooxygenase (COX), cross-react with each other in causing respiratory reactions, often upon first exposure to the new NSAID. Furthermore, respiratory reactions are dose dependent, so that while small doses of ASA or other NSAIDs may not induce reactions, larger doses of these COX-inhibiting drugs can induce progressively more severe respiratory reactions.

Definition of ASA-Sensitive Respiratory Disease

Sensitivity to ASA and other NSAIDs occurs in patients with chronic rhinitis, sinusitis, nasal polyps, and asthma. ASA-sensitive respiratory disease (ASRD) is defined by an underlying respiratory inflammation that starts with, and continues in the absence of, exposure to ASA/NSAIDs. Such patients can only be identified as ASA sensitive after experiencing a respiratory reaction to ASA or another NSAID. Except for their sensitivity to ASA/NSAIDs, ASA-sensitive asthmatic patients cannot be distinguished from patients with similar clinical presentations. Respiratory inflammation frequently precedes the development of ASA/NSAID-induced reactions by a number of years.

ASA sensitivity is acquired, usually in the third or fourth decades of life. Before the onset of sensitivity, all patients tolerate ASA and NSAIDs without ill effects.

Clinical Features of Aspirin-Sensitive Respiratory Disease

The typical patient with ASRD is an adult between 20 and 50 years of age. Although either sex can be afflicted with aspirin disease, the condition is slightly more common in women (56% in our series of 450 ASRD patients). After having been in good health and having uncomplicated upper respiratory tract infections (URIs) in the past, the patient characteristically develops a URI that persists and leads to chronic inflammation in the nasal and sinus membranes. The patient gradually worsens, and the condition eventually evolves into a chronic eosinophilic rhinosinusitis, usually with nasal polyps and secondary purulent pansinusitis.

The inflammatory disease may be limited to the upper airway, but more commonly lower respiratory tract inflammation eventually appears. This "intrinsic" type of asthma progresses, frequently requires corticosteroids to maintain bronchial or nasal function, and usually becomes complicated by intractable pansinusitis. Samter was the first to describe the classic ASA triad, consisting of rhinitis with nasal polyps, asthma, and ASA sensitivity (1).

Because these patients are frequently treated with topical corticosteroids, nasal cytograms may not contain eosinophils. Peripheral blood eosinophilia tends to be elevated, unless systemic corticosteroids are used. Anosmia is present in most patients with ASA respiratory disease. Roentgenographic abnormalities, detected by either plain roentgenograms or CT scans, are expected. As the disease progresses, the sinuses become more opacified and usually evolve into pansinusitis. In 234 asthmatic patients who were referred to the Scripps Clinic for aspirin desensitization between 1991 and 1997, 200 were proven to be ASA sensitive, using oral challenges with ASA. We could not obtain documentation of previous sinus x-rays or CAT scans in 6 patients. In the remaining 194 patients, 187 (96%) had abnormal sinus opacifications detected by sinus x-rays or CAT scans. Of further interest, 172 of 194 (89%) in this group of selected ASRD patients had previously undergone sinus/polyp surgery. From a diagnostic viewpoint, an asthmatic patient who cannot smell, has nasal polyps and abnormal sinus x-rays, and has undergone previous sinus surgery is a likely candidate for ASA respiratory sensitivity.

Prevalence of Aspirin-Sensitive Respiratory Disease

The prevalence of ASA-sensitive asthma varies, depending on the study population and the methods used to detect and report such individuals (2). Some reports present prevalence data based solely upon patient history of reactions to ASA. Such studies underestimate ASA sensitivity, because many patients cannot correlate an asthma attack with ASA or NSAID ingestion or have avoided ASA/NSAIDs entirely. Reports from tertiary referral centers where prospective oral ASA challenges were performed detected the following prevalence of ASA-sensitive asthmatic patients: In a 1972 study conducted at Scripps Clinic and Research Foundation, 9% of consecutive adult asthmatic patients challenged with oral ASA were found to be ASA sensitive. At the National Jewish Hospital in Denver, 20% of the adult asthmatic population was found to have ASA respiratory sensitivity. These prevalence data are for all asthmatic patients without any screening for specific clinical characteristics (2).

The prevalence of ASA sensitivity in asthmatic patients with associated rhinosinusitis and/or nasal polyps, without a history of ASA-induced respiratory reactions, was 30% to 40%. Adult asthmatic patients who reported a previous history of ASA-induced respiratory reaction had an incidence of positive oral ASA challenges ranging between 66% and 97% (2).

Currently there are no guidelines on which asthmatic patients should be warned to avoid ASA and NSAIDs. Obviously, those who have experienced a respiratory reaction to one NSAID should be warned to avoid all NSAIDs, including ASA. For patients with rhinosinusits and aggressive nasal polyp formation, it is unknown whether a reaction will occur until an NSAID is ingested. In fact, there is no *in vitro* test that can identify such patients. Therefore because there is a 30% to 40% chance of ASA/NSAID sensitivity in patients with nasal polyps and asthma, many physicians warn this subset of asthmatics to avoid ASA and NSAIDs. Asthmatic patients who are already taking, or have taken, ASA or one of the NSAIDs in the past 2 months without adverse effect cannot have ASRD at that point in time. Asthmatic patients without nasal polyposis are at low risk for reaction to ASA/NSAIDs (10%), and most physicians do not warn these patients to avoid ASA and NSAIDs.

Mechanisms

Aspirin-Sensitive Respiratory Disease

Mechanisms that account for underlying ASA respiratory disease or respiratory reactions to ASA have been partly clarified. Vanselow and Smith were the first to report a cross-reaction between ASA and indomethacin in 1967.

This observation has been confirmed by every subsequent investigator and is now recognized to be an irrefutable fact (1,3). Immune recognition of ASA and the widely different chemical structures of the NSAIDs is unlikely, and first-exposure reactions to NSAIDs occur routinely, eliminating any possibility of previous immune sensitization. Furthermore, IgE antibodies to ASA or NSAIDs have not been demonstrated in ASRD patients.

In 1971, Vane discovered the shared pharmacologic effect of ASA and NSAIDs, namely the inhibition of cyclooxygenase in the metabolic cascade of arachidonic acid metabolism (4). With the discovery by Samuelsson in the early 1980s of a second metabolic pathway (5-lipoxygenase), which synthesizes leukotrienes (5), it became apparent that arachidonate could be preferentially diverted down the 5-lipoxygenase pathway when the primary cyclooxygenase pathway was blocked. The 5-lipoxygenase products, or leukotrienes, mediate chemotaxis (LTB_4) and are also potent mediators of bronchoconstriction, vasodilation, attraction of eosinophils, and mucus secretion (LTC_4, LTD_4, and LTE_4) (5).

Figure 13-1 summarizes our understanding of the pathogenesis of ASRD, ASA/NSAID induced reactions, and ASA desensitization:

- *Baseline (Before ASA is Introduced)*—Increased numbers of activated mast cells and eosinophils are present in respiratory mucosa in ASRD patients. Both 5-LO and the COX-1 and 2 pathways are actively synthesizing inflammatory products. A partial brake on 5-LO and granules is provided by PGE_2, which is synthesized via COX-1 and 2.

- *Aspirin/NSAID Induced Reactions*—COX-1 is destroyed by ASA and synthesis of PGE2 abruptly ceases. Because this pathway is the major source of PGE_2, the brake on 5-LO and granules is released, allowing a surge in synthesis of new leukotrienes and the extrusion of histamine/tryptase granules. Cyst-LT_1 receptors on bronchi, blood vessels, and mucous glands (not shown) are up-regulated and respond to the flood of LTs, producing forceful and prolonged bronchospasm, vasodilation with edema formation, mucous secretion, and recruitment of additional eosinophils.

- *Aspirin Desensitization*—COX-1 and COX-2 are disabled, and no further synthesis of prostanoids occurs. LT synthesis returns to baseline, and cyst-LT_1 receptors are down-regulated in their response to LTs. Histamine is no longer released from granules.

All biochemical events shown in Figure 13-1 occur within mast cells with terminal LTs, prostanoids, histamine, and tryptase, leaving the mast cells to affect target receptors. CysLT$_1$-receptors are present on target cells: bronchial smooth muscle (bronchoconstriction), mucous glands (secretion of mucus), peribronchial venules (leakage of plasma with edema), and eosinophils (chemoatractants). The lower respiratory reactions to ASA in ASRD patients can largely be explained by LTs stimulating cysLT$_1$-receptors. Upper airway reactions are caused by LTs and histamine.

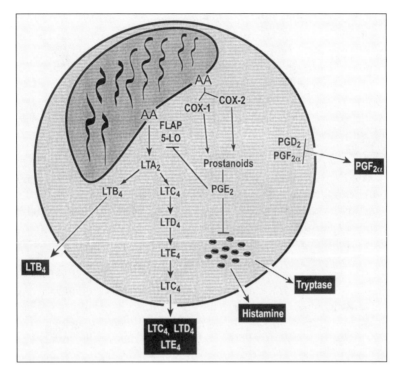

Figure 13-1   Respiratory mucosal mast cell. See text for discussion.

Mast cells and eosinophils, infiltrating nasal and bronchial mucosa, synthesize arachidonic products. Eosinophils release major basic protein (MBP) and eosinophil cationic protein (ECP). Mast cells release preformed granule-associated mediators (histamine and tryptase). Mast cells and eosinophils have been observed within the nasal cytograms, nasal tissue biopsies, bronchial biopsies, and bronchoalveolar lavage fluid (BALF) taken from ASA-sensitive asthmatic patients. In ASA-sensitive asthmatics, BALF contains increased numbers of eosinophils and eosinophil cationic protein when compared with the bronchial alveolar lavage fluid from control asthmatics. Furthermore, BALF contained increased concentrations of LTs before introduction of ASA-lysine (2). Urine sampling in ASA-sensitive asthmatics, when compared with control asthmatics and normals, shows higher levels of baseline LTE_4 and thromboxane B_2 (2,6).

Szczeklik (7) has suggested that ASA disease is a chronic or latent viral infection of the respiratory mucosa. The onset of ASA disease, following a viral URI, is compatible with his hypothesis. Activated T lymphocytes or other cells, in the absence of negative feedback, secrete excessive quantities of cytokines and chemokines. These in turn up-regulate genes, via transcription factors, and synthesize inflammatory enzymes (e.g., LTC_4 synthase) in mast cells and eosinophils.

Aspirin/NSAID Induced Respiratory Reactions

Although a mast cell is depicted in Figure 13-1, similar arachidonate metabolism also occurs in other inflammatory cells, including eosinophils. Two COX molecules have been identified. COX-1 is constantly synthesized in most mammalian cells (constitutive form), and its products regulate many physiologic functions (PGE_2, for example, is protective of gut mucosa). A second isoform is COX-2, which is restricted to inflammatory cells and induced during inflammation. ASA and most NSAIDs inhibit both COX-1 and COX-2. Dexamethasone interferes with transcription factors and decreases synthesis of COX-2. Selective COX-2 inhibitor drugs only fill the COX channel of COX-2 (their chemical configuration prevents them from entering the COX-1 channel and inhibiting the function of COX-1).

The bulk of the evidence indicates that inhibition of COX-1 is the inciting event in ASA-induced respiratory reactions (see Fig. 13-1). ASA and NSAIDs rapidly acetylate (ASA) or bind (NSAID) to COX-1, immediately preventing synthesis of COX products, including PGE_2. This releases the inhibitory effects of PGE_2 on the 5-LO enzymes and mast cell granular release mechanisms. At the same time arachidonic acid synthesis continues, preferentially driving arachidonate molecules down the 5-LO pathway. The lower respiratory reaction is largely caused by leukotrienes.

Histamine and tryptase are also released from mast cells during ASA- or NSAID-induced respiratory reactions, and histamine appears to have a significant role in causing rhinitis and conjunctivitis, as well as in flushing and urticaria (2).

Desensitization with Acetylsalicylic Acid

The term *desensitization* is usually used to describe an alteration in immune responses engineered by repeated exposure to injected antigens, thus reducing IgE-mediated reactions (see Chapter 8). Because IgE-mediated mechanisms have nothing to do with ASA respiratory sensitivity, desensitization is used here in its broadest sense.

In 1980, Stevenson and co-workers reported two ASA-sensitive asthmatics who became refractory to ASA after single blind oral challenges with ASA. After first achieving ASA desensitization, both patients experienced improvement in respiratory disease activity when they were treated with daily ASA. All ASA-sensitive asthmatics are capable of undergoing desensitization to ASA (2). Since 1980, we have successfully desensitized 620 consecutive ASA sensitive patients. After ASA desensitization, in the absence of further exposure to ASA, the desensitized state persists for 2 to 5 days, with full sensitivity returning after withholding ASA for 7 days. Also, cross-desensitization between ASA and any of the NSAIDs that inhibit COX-1 also occurs. During oral ASA challenges, desensitization is accomplished by reintroducing the dose of ASA that initiated the ASA reaction on the previous day. If there is no reaction to the same dose, the next highest dose is

Table 13-1 Single-Blind Three-Day Oral Aspirin (ASA) Challenge, Followed by Aspirin Desensitization*

Time	Day 1	Day 2	Day 3
7:00 A.M.	Placebo	ASA 30 mg	ASA 100–150 mg
10:00 A.M.	Placebo	ASA 45–60 mg	ASA 150–325 mg
1:00 P.M.	Placebo	ASA 60–100 mg	ASA 325–650 mg

* FEV_1 values were obtained by spirometry every hour during challenges. A 15% or more decline in FEV_1 value combined with a naso-ocular reaction is evidence of a respiratory reaction.

Individualized by the physician, both with respect to incremental increases and ASA dosage and timing of administration of each dose.

Desensitization: After respiratory reaction, treat and wait until reaction resolves. Repeat same challenge dose of ASA until no reaction occurs, then advance to the next dose. Continue this course until reaching a dose of 650 mg, at which time desensitization is completed.

given and repeated until further reactions cease (Table 13-1). This process of escalating doses of ASA continues until the patient can tolerate 650 mg of ASA without any reactions. ASA challenges and desensitization should be performed by board-certified allergists and immunologists or pulmonary specialists, who are experienced with this procedure and are prepared to treat severe asthma attacks. Patients must be monitored closely with pulmonary function tests performed every hour and at the first sign of a respiratory reaction. Close nursing observation and care, along with all treatment modalities, must be available.

Candidates for ASA desensitization are

1. Patients with coronary artery disease, who need ASA for prophylaxis

2. Patients with arthritis, particularly those who are unresponsive to other treatments

3. Patients with ASRD who have intractable nasal polyp formation and sinusitis

Eight studies have reported on the clinical efficacy of ASA desensitization followed by daily ASA treatment (2). In the most recent study, 65 ASA-sensitive asthmatic patients were treated with ASA 650 mg bid after ASA desensitization. The clinical courses before and after 1 to 6 years of daily ASA treatment were compared (8). While the patients were under treatment with ASA, objective clinical criteria demonstrated significant improvement in their clinical courses, particularly a reduction in sinusitis. Simultaneously, requirements for systemic corticosteroids declined significantly.

The pathogenesis of aspirin desensitization is largely unknown. During acute desensitization, defined as normal lung function 3 hr after the first ingestion of ASA, histamine and LTC_4 disappeared in nasal secretions and urine LTE_4 declined to similar levels found in baseline specimens (9). In long-term aspirin desensitization after treatment with aspirin 650 mg twice a day for at least 2 weeks, LTB_4 synthesis in monocytes declined substantially to the same levels as found in normal controls (2). Such experiments suggest that aspirin desensitization, particularly long-term treatment with higher doses of aspirin, inhibits COX-1 and COX-2 and may down-regulate cyst-LT_1 receptors in smooth muscles, vascular endothelium, and inflammatory cells.

Cross-Reactions and Cross-Desensitization

Strong Inhibitors of COX-1 and Weak Inhibitors of COX-2
All NSAIDs that inhibit COX-1 *in vitro* cross-react with ASA, inducing the respiratory reactions described above (Table 13-2) and also participate in cross-desensitization. All the NSAIDs in this category also inhibit COX-2 but usually at 50 to 100 times the concentration of the NSAID required to inhibit COX-1. The average ASA threshold dose of 60 mg, which induces a respiratory reaction, is too small to inhibit COX-2.

Weak Inhibitors of COX-1 and Little or No Effect on COX-2
Cross-reactivity between ASA and compounds that are weak inhibitors of COX-1, and have no or minimal effect on COX-2, such as acetaminophen and salsalate, is also of interest. One would assume that weak inhibitors of COX-1 would clinically cross-react poorly, if at all, with ASA, because of the evidence that COX-1 inhibition is the initiating event in ASA-induced respiratory reactions.

ACETAMINOPHEN
Initial studies reported a low-to-absent rate of cross-reactivity between acetaminophen and ASA. In these studies, however, oral challenges were performed with doses of acetaminophen equal to or less than 650 mg. In a large study of 50 known ASA-sensitive asthmatics, using a challenge dose

Table 13-2   Nonsteroidal Anti-Inflammatory Drugs That Inhibit COX-1 and Cross-React with Aspirin 100% of the Time

Generic Name	Trade Name	Generic Name	Trade Name
Piroxicam	Feldene	Mefenamic acid	Ponstel
Indomethacin	Indocin	Flurbiprofen	Ansaid
Sulindac	Clinoril	Diflunisal	Dolobid
Tolmetin	Tolectin	Ketoprofen	Orudis, Oruvail
Ibuprofen	Motrin, Rufen, Advil	Diclofenac	Voltaren
Naproxen	Naprosyn, Alleve	Ketoralac	Toradol
Naproxen sodium	Anaprox	Etodolac	Lodine
Fenoprofen	Nalfon	Nabumetone	Relafen
Meclofenamate	Meclomen	Oxaprozin	Daypro

of acetaminophen 1000 mg and then 1500 mg, respiratory reactions were reported in 34% of the study subjects (10). The respiratory reactions were generally mild, easily treated, and only occurred in a minority of ASA-sensitive asthmatics.

SALSALATE

Salsalate is a partly effective anti-inflammatory agent that is used in the treatment of arthritis. Salsalate is a weak inhibitor of COX-1. Stevenson et al (11) studied 10 ASA-sensitive asthmatics to evaluate cross-sensitivity to salsalate. Two of the 10 experienced bronchospastic reactions but only when 2 g of the drug were ingested. Repeat challenges with 2 g of salsalate reproduced the same reactions. Both patients then underwent ASA challenge and desensitization. Once desensitized to ASA, both patients were able to ingest 2 g of salsalate without adverse reactions, demonstrating cross-desensitization. Salsalate, a weak inhibitor of COX-1, behaves like ASA and NSAIDs in producing respiratory reactions but only when large doses are ingested and only in a minority of ASA-sensitive asthmatics.

Partially Selective COX-2 Inhibitors That Also Inhibit COX-1 at Higher Concentrations

Meloxicam (Mobic), marketed in the United States, and nimsulide, marketed in Europe and South America, are interesting NSAIDs because they fall into a different inhibition category. They preferentially inhibit COX-2 but, as the doses of these drugs are increased, they begin to inhibit COX-1 also. However, unlike the NSAIDs listed in Table 13-1, these two drugs are very weak inhibitors of COX-1, even at high concentrations. Considerable experience with these drugs in Europe and South America indicates that in standard doses meloxicam and nimsulide do not participate in respiratory cross-reactions with ASA. However, after increasing the doses of these anti-inflammatory drugs, a small percentage of ASA-sensitive asthmatic patients experience very mild respiratory reactions.

Selective COX-2 Inhibitors

Two selective inhibitors of COX-2 were released in the United States in the spring of 1999. These anti-arthritis drugs, celecoxib (Celebrex) and rofecoxib (Vioxx), are unique in that they selectively inhibit COX-2 without affecting COX-1, even when given in higher concentrations. Therefore, from the moment of their introduction, there was no reason to believe that they would cause respiratory reactions in ASA-sensitive asthmatics. However, because there were no data to support this hypothesis, both pharmaceutical companies provided warning labels that recommended that these drugs should be withheld from ASA-sensitive asthmatics and should be given with great caution to any asthmatic patients.

At the Scripps Clinic, we have studied many ASA-sensitive asthmatics to determine whether or not cross-reactivity with selective COX-2 inhibitors might occur. As of January 2002, we have challenged 60 ASRD patients with rofecoxib and no adverse effects have occurred. Statistically, cross-reactivity between rofecoxib and ASA will not occur in the larger population of ASA-sensitive asthmatic subjects. We have challenged 60 ASA-sensitive asthmatics with celecoxib and none has reacted.

Cross-reactivity between selective COX-2 inhibitors and ASA does not appear to occur. This fact does not prevent COX-2 inhibitors from inducing other types of reactions.

Noninhibitors of COX-1 or COX-2

Some authors have reported that other chemicals, dyes, and additives also cause respiratory reactions in ASA-sensitive asthmatics, even though these compounds do not inhibit COX-1 or COX-2. Such chemicals include azo and nonazo dyes, sulfites, monosodium glutamate, benzoates, and hydrocortisone succinate. At the Scripps Clinic extensive oral challenges have been performed with these chemicals in ASA-sensitive asthmatics and respiratory reactions have not occurred. At this time, most investigators in this field join us in expressing serious doubts that there is any cross-reactivity between ASA and chemicals that do not inhibit COX-1.

The best known azo dye is Yellow #5 (tartrazine) because it has been promoted by some authors to be responsible for cross-sensitivity reactions with ASA (1). When reviewing these publications, where an apparent cross-sensitivity has been reported, one is struck by the fact that earlier studies were conducted when patient airways were unstable and anti-asthmatic therapy had been simultaneously withdrawn. In the largest study of tartrazine and ASA sensitivity, Stevenson et al (12) challenged 150 known ASA-sensitive asthmatics with tartrazine 25 and 50 mg. Six (4%) experienced a 20% or more decrease in FEV_1 values during open screening challenges with tartrazine. All repeat challenges with tartrazine, using the same dose associated with declining FEV_1 values in the screening challenges, were negative during double-blind follow-up oral challenges with tartrazine. Tartrazine has not been shown to inhibit COX-1 or COX-2 *in vitro* and therefore would not be expected to cross-react with ASA and NSAIDs.

Aspirin-Sensitive Respiratory Disease and Leukotriene Modifiers

Theoretically, drugs that either inhibit or antagonize LTs should be effective in protecting ASA-sensitive asthmatics from inadvertent exposure to ASA/NSAIDs. With respect to protection, current literature review demonstrates that LT modifiers might protect patients from bronchospasm during oral and inhalation ASA challenges when small provoking doses of ASA are used (usually 60 mg of ASA orally). Unfortunately, protection is inconsistent after ingesting small ASA doses and inadequate in preventing ASRD patients from respiratory reactions after exposure to larger (therapeutic) doses of ASA or other NSAIDs. Reports have described ASA-sensitive asthmatics who experienced spontaneous asthma attacks after inadvertent exposure to full therapeutic doses of ASA or one of the NSAIDs while taking zileuton (Zyflo).

At the Scripps Clinic we challenged six known ASA-sensitive asthmatics with ASA and all reacted. They were then treated with zileuton 600 mg qid and re-challenged with ASA. One patient was not protected at all by zileuton, reacting with a 53% drop in FEV_1 value after ingesting 45 mg of ASA. The other five patients also reacted to ASA but, after zyleuton protection, their asthmatic responses were less severe and the doses required to induce the reactions were higher.

Respiratory reactions to ASA and NSAIDs during ongoing treatment with zafirlukast (Accolate) and montelukast (Singulair) have been reported. A second study at Scripps Clinic involved ten ASRD patients, pretreated with montelukast (14). Half converted from bronchospastic and naso-ocular reactions, during their baseline reactions without montelukast protection, to naso-ocular reactions only, with montelukast protection. However, four patients experienced the same degree of bronchospastic responses to ASA that they had experienced without montelukast protection. Thus the theoretical advantages of treatment with LT-modifying drugs does not include protection from inadvertent exposure to NSAIDs in ASA-sensitive asthmatic patients.

With respect to whether ASRD patients should be treated with LT-modifying drugs for control of the underlying disease, there is still some controversy. Although short-term studies, using treatment with either zileuton or montelukast, show a positive effect on asthma control, the differences are not spectacular. Those of us who care for large numbers of ASRD patients are impressed by the variability of response to LT modifiers in patients who theoretically should all have excessive synthesis of LTs and impressive responses to LT modifiers. Yet this is not the case. Only about half of ASRD patients respond impressively to LT modifier therapy. For reasons that are unclear, half of ASRD patients do not improve with LT modifier therapy.

Case 13-1 is that of a patient with asthma induced by aspirin.

Beta-Adrenergic Blocker Induced Asthma

Clinical Features

Shortly after the introduction of beta-adrenergic receptor antagonists in the 1960s, reports of worsening of asthma in asthmatic patients treated with these drugs began to appear. For the most part, a dose-dependent effect seemed to predominate in reported cases, with some milder asthmatic patients actually being able to tolerate low doses of beta-blockers without apparent adverse effects on their asthma. The precipitated asthma is generally described as a "troublesome" attack rather than as an acute one. However, there are reports of severe asthma exacerbations in patients with mild asthma occurring shortly after starting beta-blocker therapy. Even beta-blocker eye

---

CASE 13-1   *Patient with asthma induced by aspirin*

A 42-year-old male developed a viral URI and persisting symptoms of nasal congestion. He then developed wheezing for the first time. Nasal congestion and anosmia continued, and he sought help from an ENT specialist. This physician obtained a sinus CT scan and found polyps and pansinusitis. A sinus operation was performed, but the polyps grew back. One day the patient took 2 ibuprofen tablets for a headache. Forty five minutes later, his nose began to run and he started to wheeze and become short of breath. His wife insisted on taking him to the emergency room, where he was treated with inhaled bronchodilators and sent home 4 hr later. He was told to avoid aspirin and NSAIDs.

A year later he was admitted to the hospital for shoulder surgery. He told the orthopedic surgeon that he was allergic to aspirin and NSAIDs. The surgeon said that everything would be all right because he would be treating the patient with Percodan. Post-operatively, the patient received his first Percodan tablet and 45 min later began to have profuse rhinorrhea and severe asthma. Respiratory therapy was called for, and the patient received eight treatments with nebulized albuterol over the next 4 hr. All his symptoms cleared at that point and he said he felt "great." His nose congestion was gone, and he could smell a little.

The patient confronted his surgeon the next morning, saying that he suspected that ibuprofen was in the Percodan. The surgeon insisted that there was no ibuprofen in the Percodan and encouraged the patient to continue to take it for pain. That day the patient received the Percodan, did not have a reaction, and felt great all day. He was discharged from the hospital the next day, feeling fine, able to smell, and without any asthma. The patient concluded that the orthopedic surgeon was a great doctor for operating successfully and knowing how to manage his pain medicines.

Discussion

Percodan contains 325 mg of ASA and 4.5 mg of oxycodone. The orthopedist caused a serious asthma reaction by prescribing ASA (Percodan). Following the reaction to ASA 325 mg, the patient was desensitized to aspirin, which was also beginning to effectively decrease his nasal congestion. No further reactions to Percodan occurred because the patient was in the ASA-desensitized state. If, however, the patient had received another dose of Percodan 7 or more days later, he would have had the same severe respiratory reaction.

---

drops, used to treat glaucoma, have precipitated severe asthma attacks. Death has occurred during some of these beta-blocker induced asthma attacks (Case 13-2).

Nonselective beta-adrenergic antagonists, which block beta$_1$-receptors in the heart and blood vessels as well as beta$_2$-receptors on bronchial smooth muscles, are propranolol (Inderal), sotalol (Betapace), timolol (Blocadren), and nadolol. Selective beta$_1$-adrenergic receptor blocking agents are atenolol (Tenormin), metoprolol (Toprol), betaxolol (Kerlone),

> **CASE 13-2**   *Fatal beta-blocker asthma attack in an 18-year-old girl*
>
> An 18-year-old girl had mild asthma caused by allergy to house dust. She was treated with daily fluticasone 110 2 puffs bid and infrequent use of an albuterol inhaler. One afternoon she developed a severe migraine. Her mother called the family physician, who had just attended a CME course during which the use of propranolol in treatment of migraines had been discussed. Over the telephone the family physician prescribed Inderal (propranolol) 40 mg q 6 hr until the migraine was gone.
>
> The girl's mother obtained the prescription and gave her daughter the first dose of 40 mg of Inderal. An hour later, the girl began having asthma that soon became more severe. She used her albuterol inhaler and nothing happened. The parents rushed her to the emergency room (20 minutes away). The girl turned blue and lost consciousness on the way to the hospital. Their only daughter was dead on arrival.
>
> **Discussion**
>
> Sometimes a little learning is a dangerous thing. Though beta-blockers seem to work as prophylaxis in some patients with migraine, they are generally not effective for fully developed migraine attacks. Therefore one of the tragedies in this case is that the wrong migraine therapy was prescribed in the first place.
>
> Irrespective of their use in other conditions, beta-blockers are contraindicated in asthmatics. Although the case of this young asthmatic patient was unusual, beta-blockers can cause severe asthma attacks in people with mild persistent asthma.

and bisoprolol (Zebeta); these preferentially block beta$_1$-receptors in the heart. At higher doses of these "selective" blockers, beta$_2$-blockade begins to occur and becomes more pronounced as the doses of these drugs are increased. However, for the most part, nonselective beta-adrenergic antagonists are more likely to induce asthma in known asthmatics than are the selective beta$_1$-adrenergic antagonists, particularly when the selective beta$_1$-blockers are used in lower doses. In addition, asthma that has been induced by low-dose beta$_1$-adrenergic receptor antagonists can generally be reversed more easily with a beta$_2$-agonist than if nonselective beta-adrenergic blockers are in use. However, this reversal cannot be counted upon with nonselective adrenergic blocker therapy or even with high-dose beta$_1$-blocker therapy. Fortunately, after discontinuing beta-blockers, all asthmatics should revert to their former level of asthma activity. It is recommended that all beta-blockers be withheld from asthmatic patients.

Mechanisms

The mechanism through which beta-blockers induce asthma is not entirely clear. The evidence that beta-blockers cause the disease called *chronic asthma* has never been substantiated. There are two leading theories that explain the effects of beta-adrenergic antagonists on asthmatic airways. The first theory is related to mast cells. *In vitro* experiments have shown that IgE-mediated release of histamine from human lung mast cells can be inhibited by adding a beta$_2$-agonist, salmeterol. Thus the addition of a nonspecific beta-blocker might prevent catecholamine stabilization of mast cells. In support of this theory is the fact that pretreatment with cromolyn sodium, a mast cell stabilizer, prevents the bronchoconstriction normally induced by propranolol in asthmatic subjects.

A second theory is related to the fact that cholinergic nerves in human airways contain beta$_2$-receptors as a feedback mechanism for decreasing release of acetyl choline (Fig. 13-2). When blocked by a beta-receptor antagonist, acetyl choline accumulates in the cholinergic nerves, with stimulation of smooth muscle constriction via cholinergic receptors on the bronchial smooth muscles (15).

Angiotensin-Converting Enzyme Inhibitors and Asthma

A popular class of drugs called *angiotensin converting enzyme* (ACE) inhibitors has been developed for the treatment of hypertension. These drugs include quinapril (Accupril), perindopril (Aceon), ramipril (Altace), captopril, benazepril (Lotensin), trandolapril (Mavik), fosinopril (Monopril), lisinopril (Prinivil, Zestril), moexipril (Univasc), and enalapril (Vasotec).

Drugs that inhibit ACE enhance accumulation of bradykininase, an enzyme that normally degrades bradykinin in the lung. Bradykinin, an active bronchoconstrictor and vasodilator, has the potential to induce asthma. However, lung tissue is rich in kininases that destroy bradykinin very rapidly, even in the absence of ACE. Therefore precisely how ACE inhibitors accumulate in bronchial tissues and cause asthma attacks is not entirely clear.

Concomitantly, about 10% of patients treated with an ACE inhibitor develop angioedema and another 20% develop a nonproductive annoying cough. Both of these side effects are reversed by discontinuing the responsible ACE inhibitor drug. It is assumed that formation of kinins initiates both angioedema and cough. If the ACE inhibitor can cause angioedema and cough, the logical extension of this argument proposes the theory that the ACE inhibitor can also induce bronchospasm (15).

What is the evidence that an ACE inhibitor can cause bronchospasm? One retrospective study showed that asthma was twice as common in patients treated with an ACE inhibitor than in a matched control group treated with a lipid-lowering drug. In a controlled trial in asthmatics (with and without cough) who also had hypertension, there was no change in lung function or cough after administering captopril. Furthermore, there was no increase in bronchial reactivity to inhalation of histamine or bradykinin in

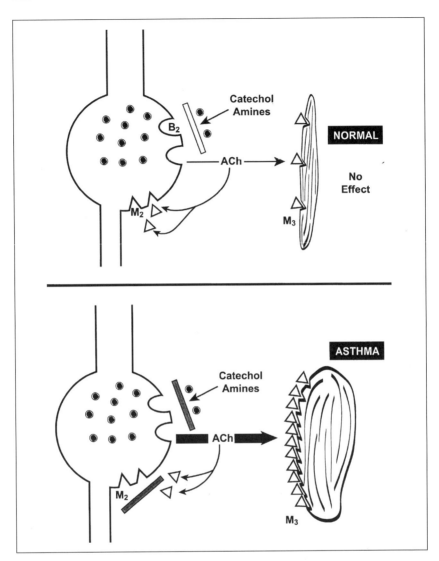

Figure 13-2   Cholinergic nerve ending. *Top*, Normal cholinergic nerve ending. Beta$_2$-receptors receive catecholamines, which signal a reduction in release of acetylcholine (ACh). Even with blockade of beta$_2$-receptors by beta-blocking drugs, the alternative M$_2$ feedback loop is intact. Thus as ACh is secreted it stimulates muscarinic receptors to signal a reduction in secretion of further ACh molecules. ACh is never allowed to increase in concentration. At the same time, bronchial smooth muscles also have fewer M$_3$-receptors to receive ACh molecules. *Bottom*, Cholinergic nerve ending from an asthmatic patient. For reasons not entirely clear, M$_2$-receptors are partially or completely blocked in asthmatics. Also, bronchial smooth muscles are hypertrophic and M$_3$-receptors are increased in number. Therefore, when beta$_2$-receptors are blocked, the alternative feedback loop is not available and increased ACh is secreted. Stimulation of M$_3$-receptors on bronchial smooth muscles occurs, leading to cholinergic bronchospasm.

asthmatic patients pretreated with captopril. In a group of 21 asthmatic patients given an ACE inhibitor (enalapril 10 to 20 mg qid) for 3 weeks, 3 patients developed a cough and 1 patient developed wheezing during this short-term trial. All patients, including these 4 patients, had normal lung function studies before, during, and after the trial. PD_{20} to methacholine inhalation was unchanged while taking the ACE inhbitor in all 21 patients, including the 3 coughing patients and the one with mild "wheezing" (15).

All of these studies point toward the conclusion that ACE inhibitors do not induce fundamental biochemical or mediator changes that worsen asthmatic activity in most asthmatic patients. Furthermore, ACE inhibitor induced angioedema or cough does not appear to predispose an asthmatic or a nonasthmatic individual to experience bronchospastic reactions to ACE inhibitors (15). On the other hand, there may be asthmatic patients whose asthma is worsened by ACE inhibitors. In such individuals, other anti-hypertensive drugs should be used. A definitive study is sorely needed.

REFERENCES

1. **Samter M, Beers R Jr.** Intolerance to aspirin: clinical studies and consideration of its pathogenesis. Ann Intern Med. 1968;68:975–83.

2. **Stevenson DD, Simon RA.** Sensitivity to aspirin and nonsteroidal antiinflammatory drugs. In: Middleton EJ, Reed CE, Ellis EF, et al. Allergy: Principles and Practice, 5th ed. St. Louis: CV Mosby; 1998:1225–34.

3. **Vanselow NA, Smith JR.** Bronchial asthma induced by indomethacin. Ann Intern Med. 1967;66:568–73.

4. **Vane JR.** Inhibition of prostaglandin synthesis as a mechanism of action for aspirin-like drugs. Nature New Biol. 1971;231:232–5.

5. **Samuelsson B, Hammarstroem S, Murphy RC, et al.** Leukotrienes and slow reacting substance of anaphylaxis (SRS-A). Allergy. 1980;35:375–81.

6. **Szczeklik A, Sladek K, Dworski R, et al.** Bronchial aspirin challenge causes specific eicosanoid response in aspirin-sensitive asthmatics. Am J Crit Care Med. 1996;154:1608–14.

7. **Szczeklik A.** The cyclooxygenase theory of aspirin-induced asthma [Review]. Eur Resp J. 1990;3:588–93.

8. **Stevenson DD, Hankammer MA, Mathison DA, et al.** Aspirin desensitization treatment of aspirin sensitive rhinosinusitic-asthmatic patients: long-term outcomes. J Allergy Clin Immunol. 1996;98:751–8.

9. **Daffern PJ, Muilenburg D, Hugli TE, Stevenson DD.** Association of urinary leukotriene E4 excretion during oral aspirin challenges with severity of respiratory responses. J Allergy Clin Immunol. 1999;104:559–64.

10. **Settipane RA, Stevenson DD.** Prevalence of acetaminophen cross-sensitivity in aspirin-sensitive asthmatic patients. J Allergy Clin Immunol. 1995;96:480–5.

11. **Stevenson DD, Hougham A, Schrank P, et al.** Disalcid cross-sensitivity in aspirin-sensitive asthmatics. J Allergy Clin Immunol. 1990;86:749–58.

12. **Stevenson DD, Simon RA, Lumry WR, Mathison DA.** Adverse reactions to tartrazine. J Allergy Clin Immunol. 1986;78:182–91.

13. **Pauls JD, Simon RA, Daffern PJ, Stevenson DD.** Lack of effect of the 5-lipoxy-genase inhibitor zileuton in blocking oral aspirin challenges in aspirin-sensitive asthmatics. Ann Allergy Asthma Immunol. 2000;85:1–6.

14. **Stevenson DD, Simon RA, Mathison DA, Christiansen SC.** Montelukast is only partially effective in inhibiting aspirin responses in aspirin-sensitive asthmatics. Ann Allergy Asthma Immunol. 2000;85:477–82.

15. **Barnes,PJ.** Drug-induced asthma. In: Barnes PJ, Grunstein MM, Leff AR, Woolcock AJ, eds. Asthma. Philadelphia: Lippincott-Raven; 1997:1245–9.

14

∷ ∷ ∷

Gastroesophageal Reflux Disease and Asthma

Demetrios S. Theodoropoulos, MD, DSc

astroesophageal reflux disease (GERD) and asthma are common diseases whose concurrence is observed more frequently than accounted for by chance. Three to ten percent of the adult world population has asthma. Seven percent of the population has daily gastroesophageal reflux symptoms, and 36% of adults experience heartburn at least once a month (1). Based on these rates, the probability of an asthmatic experiencing heartburn at least once a month should not exceed 36%. Symptomatic GERD, however, is diagnosed in 45% to 89% of patients with chronic asthma (2).

The association of GERD with asthma is supported by a large number of studies, which may contribute to increased awareness among physicians and more frequent recognition of the asthma-GERD association. There is objective evidence that successful management of GERD may lead to improved control of asthma (1). Meta-analysis of 12 studies published in the last 35 years on the effects of medical anti-reflux therapy on asthma shows that treatment of GERD improves asthma symptoms in 69% and reduces the use of asthma medication in 62% of subjects. Evening peak expiratory flow rates improve in 26% of patients. The overall effect of GERD therapy on lung function, as demonstrated by spirometry, is modest but consistent in most studies. Pulmonary function tests improved in 20% to 27% of subjects after omeprazole treatment for 6 weeks or more. It appears that the effect of GERD treatment on asthma is more prominent in asthmatics with symptomatic GERD (3). This may reflect an implication of sensory nerve pathways in the pathophysiology of the asthma-GERD association or may be the result of symptom awareness and subjective improvement upon relief from GERD symptoms.

Pathophysiology

Normal intraluminal esophageal pressure range is significantly lower than gastric pressure. Reflux of gastric contents into the esophagus is only prevented by the physiological lower esophageal sphincter (LES). Although GERD is traditionally attributed to loss of the LES pressure barrier, three additional interacting factors impair the function of the LES and increase reflux: 1) esophagitis caused by the irritant effect of refluxed gastrointestinal material (gastric acid, pepsin, and bile), 2) ineffective esophageal clearing, and 3) delayed gastric emptying.

The concept of GERD as a disease comprising all four factors mentioned above is essential to an understanding of the pathophysiology and treatment of GERD. Absence of GERD implies not only an effective LES sphincter but also normal esophageal pH variations, intact esophageal mucosa, effective esophageal clearing, and regular gastric emptying. The loss of these functions during the course of GERD varies, and their restoration does not occur simultaneously when treatment is completed. Interactions between the GERD components mentioned above have practical implications. Clinical presentation may be dominated by esophageal dysmotility, resulting in delayed diagnosis. The management of GERD may be jeopardized when healing of esophagitis by acid inhibition is not immediately followed by normalization of esophageal clearing. Delayed gastric emptying may need to be addressed specifically in patients with the duodeno-gastroesophageal reflux variety of GERD, as well as those with Barrett's esophagus.

Most authors base the pathophysiology of GERD on a dynamic concept of pressure balance across the LES rather than the structural components of the LES. Many studies focus on esophageal muscular contractile responses rather than abdominal/thoracic pressure differences to explain the maintenance of pressure gradient. The importance of esophageal clearance with swallowing or during a reflux episode is emphasized. There is also increasing interest in transient lower esophageal sphincter relaxation, which occurs independently of swallowing and allows a large number of short reflux bursts usually against a background of normal sphincter tone. Both increased transient LES relaxations and impaired muscular contractile response to transient LES relaxation are recognized as GERD features and are believed to involve vagal pathways and the hindbrain.

Incompetent lower esophageal sphincter and ineffective esophageal clearing are more prevalent among patients with asthma (2). Medications used in asthma treatment promote gastroesophageal reflux in normal subjects. Theophylline decreases the LES pressure and increases acid secretion, and beta-agonists decrease the LES pressure. Steroids further impair esophageal healing. Their contribution to gastroesophageal reflux in patients with asthma is, however, moderate. Pathophysiologic changes brought about by asthma itself, such as hyperinflation and autonomic dysfunction, facilitate reflux across the LES to such an extent that discontinuation of these asthma therapies has little effect on gastroesophageal reflux (2).

Two main mechanisms have been proposed to explain the association of GERD with asthma: aspiration and neurogenic inflammation. Regurgitation followed by endotracheal aspiration is hypothesized as a mechanism causing respiratory symptoms in patients with asthma and GERD. Case reports of anesthetized patients who accidentally aspirated gastric contents and animal studies have consistently demonstrated that endotracheal aspiration precipitates responses indistiguishable from asthma exacerbation. Coughing and dyspnea can persist for a long time after a single aspiration episode. Studies using endotracheal pH monitoring show a correlation of declining mean expiratory flow with episodic endotracheal pH drop. However, studies with radioisotope meals fed to subjects with asthma and GERD, shortly before a period of recumbency, have failed to demonstrate aspiration. The negative results of these studies either reflect a poor sensitivity of the radiographic technique or indicate absence of aspiration in ambulatory subjects.

Vagally mediated reflexes resulting in neurogenic inflammation have been proposed to explain the occurrence of asthma exacerbations in the absence of aspiration. According to this model, sensory impulses originating from pain or stretch receptors in the esophagus are conveyed by the esophageal plexus of the vagus nerve to the nucleus of the solitary tract in the dorsomedial medulla, where interneurons project to the motor neuron pools in the ventrolateral medulla. From there the impulse is transmitted to motor efferents, located in the pulmonary branch of the vagus nerve, which project to the tracheobronchial tree and can cause contraction of smooth muscles, increased mucous secretion, and plasma extravasation.

The presence of acid in the esophagus causes neural enhancement of bronchial reactivity in asthmatics with GERD, as documented by studies of bronchial responsiveness to inhaled histamine, methacholine, and voluntary isocapnic hyperventilation with dry air. This effect is not observed in normal controls and is less prominent in asthmatics without GERD. Pretreatment with atropine increases the baseline maximum expiratory flow at 50% of forced vital capacity and prevents the decrease in maximum expiratory flow at 50% of forced vital capacity during esophageal acid infusion. More important is the observation that esophageal reflux alters the underlying bronchial reactivity to other stimuli. This finding has been documented by means of acid perfusion in patients with asthma but without GERD and in patients with asthma and with GERD (4). An asthmatic exposed to a second asthma trigger, therefore, has a heightened bronchoconstrictive response when repetitive reflux episodes have "sensitized" the airways.

The contribution of acid reflux to pulmonary pathophysiology is more complex than that of an additional trigger factor. The association of the two conditions is complicated by the decreased intrathoracic pressure and increased intra-abdominal pressure, caused by asthma exacerbations, which can therefore precipitate acid reflux. Thus the two diseases aggravate each other. An additional element of self-perpetuating pathology is introduced by the neural component of the asthma-GERD association. As pain signals are repeatedly generated, neural pathways undergo changes that make them more receptive to incoming pain signals and lower their threshold for generation of action potentials. Furthermore, afferent (sensory) cells in the dorsal horns, which are supposed to transmit signals in only one direction, acquire, under repetitive painful stimuli, the ability to generate additional antidromic action potentials directed backwards down the nociceptors. Pain signals from peripheral nerves, such as those innervating the lower esophagus, are heightened, and the neuropeptide effects are amplified.

Some studies explain the occurrence of GERD in asthma as a mere secondary effect of the altered intrathoracic and intra-abdominal pressures. They question whether GERD aggravates asthma and whether treatment of GERD improves asthma. These conclusions are, in most cases, based on the absence of a persistent effect of intraesophageal acid perfusion on pulmonary function tests. It can also be argued that improvement of evening peak expiratory flow after treatment for GERD in only 26% of subjects with GERD and asthma contrasts with the high prevalence (up to 89%) of GERD in asthma. These meta-analyses, however, do not appreciate the differences in efficacy between H_2-receptor antagonists and proton pump inhibitors (3,5). Furthermore, both H_2-receptor antagonists and proton pump inhibitors change the acidity of the refluxate but have a lesser effect on its volume.

The time interval between esophageal mucosal healing and restoration of normal esophageal clearing and lower esophageal sphincter pressure has not been studied. During this interval, lower esophageal distention by the nonacidic refluxate and even endotracheal aspiration continue and can affect pulmonary function in the medically treated patient. The time needed to restore normal esophageal function in the surgically treated patient is not known, but reflux of gastric fluids is blocked by fundoplication. Because retrospective studies and meta-analyses do not take these factors into account, they may underestimate the effect of GERD treatment on pulmonary function. The time interval between esophageal mucosal healing and restoration of motility may explain why most studies evaluating antireflux surgery show a marked effect of GERD treatment on pulmonary function compared with the modest effects of pharmacologic management, even though the two approaches have similar efficacy in decreasing esophageal pH and achieving mucosal healing (1). More importantly, meta-analyses published so far included data obtained from studies in which adequate acid suppression and use of effective doses of H_2-receptor antagonists/proton pump inhibitors were not demonstrated (3,5).

All limitations of meta-analyses notwithstanding, an improvement of asthma symptoms and a decrease in asthma rescue medication are estimated to occur in 69% and 62%, respectively, of asthmatics treated for GERD (3).

The effect of GERD treatment on pulmonary symptoms and function has also been recognized, at least in patients with symptomatic GERD (5).

Evaluation

Early attempts to differentiate between normal subjects experiencing clinically insignificant reflux episodes and subjects with gastroesophageal reflux disease based on frequency of symptoms helped determine the prevalence of symptoms in the general population (1). Screening of the general population for GERD symptoms is of limited diagnostic value because many patients have asymptomatic GERD and because symptom frequency and severity correlate poorly with esophageal injury. Furthermore, infrequent reflux episodes in subjects with intact clearing mechanisms are normal.

Compared with other patients with GERD, asthmatics with symptomatic GERD are easier to identify: Pulmonary symptoms are more likely than heartburn to make them seek medical attention. Furthermore, GERD symptom questionnaires may be expected to have a poor sensitivity when used in the general population but should have a high positive predictive value when used in asthmatics with GERD because positive predictive value, unlike sensitivity, is a function of prevalence. Questioning for GERD symptoms has a high yield of positive responses because of the high prevalence of GERD among asthmatics. Asthmatic subjects with symptoms such as heartburn, water brash, persistent belching, and exacerbation of heartburn or coughing when lying down shortly after meals are very likely to have GERD.

Subjects with "silent GERD" experience respiratory or airway symptoms related to GERD but do not report typical reflux symptoms. GERD in these individuals is usually diagnosed during the assessment of asthma recalcitrant to treatment or because of persistent respiratory symptoms such as nocturnal cough, sinusitis, laryngitis, and recurrent lower respiratory tract infections. Presentation is often atypical (Table 14-1). Manifestations of increased vagal tone have been reported in patients with asthma and GERD and take the form of exaggerated vasovagal responses to pain or stress stimuli (Case 14-1). The anatomic basis for the observed cardiovascular responses in patients with asthma and GERD is the innervation of all involved organs by branches of the vagal nerve, which also accounts for the original description of this nerve in the older literature as cardio-pneumo-gastric nerve. Laryngitis, sinusitis, and rhinitis have been associated with GERD (Case 14-2). These upper airway conditions may further aggravate asthma, thus mediating an additional indirect effect of GERD on asthma. Fiberoptic rhinolaryngoscopy may be useful in assessing the role of GERD in upper airway symptoms. Erythema/edema of the vocal cords, arytenoid erythema and interarytenoid thickening, posterior glottic erythema, and vocal cord scarring or ulceration have been described in patients with GERD and are attributed to the direct effects of acid exposure (1).

Table 14-1   GERD-Associated Symptoms

Gastroesophageal	Heartburn, chest/epigastric/cervical pain, water brash, belching, indigestion, nausea, vomiting, hematemesis, odynophagia, dysphagia, halitosis
Respiratory	Cough, wheeze, dyspnea
Laryngeal	Hoarseness, throat clearing, sighing dyspnea, irritation, globus, voice changes, soreness
Pharyngeal	Morning soreness, dryness, bitter taste, thirst
Nasal	Congestion, itching, sneezing, rhinorrhea
Sinus	Headache, pressure, purulent discharge
Ear	Otalgia
Dental	Loss of dental enamel
Cardiovascular	Sinus bradycardia, increased vasovagal responses
Neurologic	Opisthotonus, abnormal neck posturing, apnea
Psychological	Anorexia

Diagnosis of GERD can be based on history and a favorable response to trial with pharmacologic treatment (Fig. 14-1). A number of tests and procedures are available for the diagnosis of atypical GERD. More often these tests are used to address specific aspects of the GERD pathophysiology, management, and long-term follow-up. Ambulatory 24-hour esophageal pH monitoring is the most sensitive method for diagnosing GERD and the most effective way to demonstrate a temporal correlation of acid reflux with respiratory symptoms. The sensitivity of barium studies is not high, but demonstration of barium reflux is of high positive predictive value. Other tests may be considered depending on the specific issue at hand: clarification of symptoms (Bernstein test), ongoing esophagitis and Barrett's esophagus (endoscopy/biopsy), laryngitis (laryngoscopy), vocal cord dysfunction (flow/volume loop and laryngoscopy), assessment of peristaltic function in order to select candidates for surgery and choose operative procedure (manometry), sleep apnea (somnogram), and increased vagal output (tilt table).

Therapeutic Trial

Therapeutic trial with omeprazole 20 to 40 mg/day, lansoprazole 30 to 60 mg/day, or pantoprazole 40 mg/day for 3 months is recommended by the American Gastroenterology Association to expedite the early diagnosis of GERD in subjects with suggestive symptoms. Experience with higher doses of pantoprazole is limited. Favorable response, with decreased GERD and

CASE 14-1   *Patient with worsening of asthma symptoms and autonomic instability due to gastroesophageal reflux disease*

A 38-year-old woman with a 4-year history of mild persistent asthma presents with unexplained deterioration in her asthma control during the past year. Her main complaints are nocturnal dyspnea and cough that was not responding to albuterol and steroid inhalers. Treatment with salmeterol, three courses of oral steroids, and addition of leukotriene modifiers have not improved her symptoms. On questioning, she relates an 18-month history of retrosternal "squeezing" pain occurring at the same time as her asthma attacks. Lightheadedness, fatigue, nausea, and, on a few occasions, fainting are also reported. Her symptoms had been severe enough to prompt emergency room visits where she was evaluated several times for suspected myocardial infarction and treated for asthma exacerbation. A few electrocardiograms that she brings with her show sinus bradycardia. During her teens and early twenties she experienced two or three fainting episodes, but there had been no recurrence until a year ago. She denies heartburn, belching, epigastralgia, and vomiting, and has had no previous diagnosis of GERD. She admits to having resumed smoking, which she had previously discontinued for 10 years.

Physical examination gives measurements of 5'5", 253 lb. Blood pressure is 128/80 with a simultaneous heart rate of 44 bpm in the supine position and 98/60 with a heart rate of 50 bpm after being erect for 1 min. Climbing two flights of stairs increases her blood pressure to 138/80 and heart rate to 88/min. End expiratory wheezing is heard on forced expiration and becomes more prominent after exercise. Rhinolaryngoscopy is normal.

Esophageal manometry with acid perfusion (Bernstein test) reproduces the retrosternal pain and shows abnormal esophageal motility and hypotensive lower esophageal sphincter. Twenty-four hour, two-channel esophageal pH monitoring records 405 reflux episodes in the distal esophagus, 145 of which are postprandial, causing distal esophageal pH to drop below 4 for a total of 279 minutes (21.8% of the recorded time; upper normal limit = 3.4%). Interestingly, proximal esophageal pH recordings are within normal limits. Simultaneous Holter monitoring shows 14 bradycardic episodes, all of which follow periods of prolonged low esophageal pH. One episode of marked bradycardia with a rate of 31/min occurs during the acid perfusion test and lasts for 1.4 min. Another bradycardic episode with a rate of 28/min occurs early in the morning, with the patient recumbent, during a coughing spell and a reflux episode that lasts for 11 min.

Discussion

This patient's asthma deterioration was attributed to GERD. Her bradycardia was part of the autonomic instability with increased vagal responses characterizing some subjects with asthma-GERD association. Treatment with proton-pump inhibitors, smoking cessation, weight reduction by 10%, and regular aerobic exercise controlled the retrosternal pain. Fainting/syncope did not recur, but episodic bradycardia and postural hypotension persisted. Control of her asthma was achieved within 4 months of starting treatment with proton-pump inhibitors, with inhaled steroids twice a day and beta-agonists as needed.

CASE 14-2   *Patient with laryngitis associated with gastroesophageal reflux disease*

A 42-year-old woman who is head nurse in a busy hospital presents with asthma that is recalcitrant to treatment. Her asthma has been controlled for many years with a long-acting beta-agonist, inhaled steroids, and infrequent use of albuterol. Her past medical history was significant for peptic ulcer disease. She relates a history of frequent episodes of pharyngitis in the last few years. Review of systems reveals difficulty initiating a swallow, especially with cold fluids. On occasions she has had to use "lingual pumping" maneuvers to facilitate the swallow.

On physical examination she is slender and has a hoarse voice. She coughs and clears her throat several times during the interview. Lymphoid follicular hyperplasia (cobblestone pattern) with prominent vascularization between lymphoid follicles is noted in the posterior pharyngeal wall. Tonsils are large with deep crypts. Rhinolaryngoscopy shows erythematous vocal cords and glottis. The patient is referred for dual-channel esophageal pH monitoring, which shows a large number of reflux episodes in the distal and proximal esophagus. Esophageal motility studies are also abnormal.

Discussion

This case represents an instance of reflux laryngitis caused by proximal gastroesophageal reflux. Treatment with proton-pump inhibitors resulted in resolution of her dysphagia and cough and throat clearing. The larynx appeared normal after 6 months of GERD treatment. Her asthma was controlled with a combination of a long-acting beta-agonist and inhaled steroids.

---

respiratory symptoms and documented improvement of asthma, supports both the diagnosis of GERD and the contribution of GERD to asthma in the individual patient. Lack of response indicates that GERD is not present or is inadequately treated. Relapse of symptoms with discontinuation of the therapeutic trial supports the diagnosis of GERD. Indications for further investigation are shown in Figure 14-1.

24-Hour pH Study

Esophageal pH probe studies quantitate the exposure of esophageal mucosa to acid. They indirectly assess the integrity of the lower esophageal sphincter and the clearing ability of the esophagus. More importantly, esophageal pH probe studies with 24-hour monitoring allow a temporal correlation of reflux episodes with respiratory symptoms. The indications for pH probe studies are 1) failed therapeutic trial with proton-pump inhibitors, 2) suspected atypical GERD with predominant non-esophageal manifestations, 3) relapsing or refractory symptoms during medical treatment of GERD, 4) consideration of anti-reflux surgery in patients with

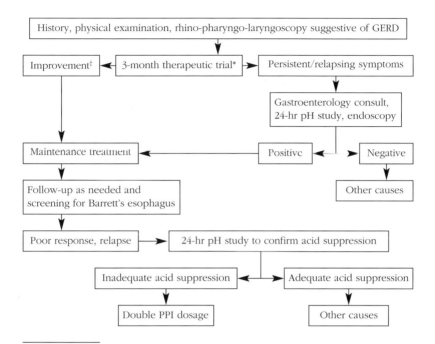

History, physical examination, rhino-pharyngo-laryngoscopy suggestive of GERD

Improvement† ◄─ 3-month therapeutic trial* ─► Persistent/relapsing symptoms

Gastroenterology consult, 24-hr pH study, endoscopy

Maintenance treatment ◄─── Positive ◄─┘ ─► Negative

Other causes

Follow-up as needed and screening for Barrett's esophagus

Poor response, relapse ─► 24-hr pH study to confirm acid suppression

Inadequate acid suppression ◄─► Adequate acid suppression

Double PPI dosage

Other causes

* Omeprazole 20–40 mg/day, lansoprazole 30–60 mg/day, pantoprazole 40 mg/day.
† Decreased use of rescue asthma medication, improved PEF rates, lowered variability of PEF rate, decreased respiratory symptoms.

Figure 14-1   Algorithm for the evaluation of GERD.

normal esophagoscopy findings, and 5) suspected reflux after anti-reflux surgery.

The specificity and accuracy of ambulatory 24-hour esophageal pH monitoring for total time with esophageal pH less than 4 to diagnose GERD are reported as 96%. When composite scores are used, which take into account multiple parameters of esophageal acid contact, the specificity and accuracy of esophageal pH monitoring may approach 100%. The parameters assessed to calculate such a composite score include: total time with pH less than 4; time of pH less than 4 when supine; time of pH less than 4 when upright; number of reflux episodes; number of reflux episodes with duration longer than 5 minutes; and duration of longest reflux episode (6). The sensitivity of esophageal pH monitoring for patients with symptomatic GERD without esophagitis may be as low as 71% (7). Absence of significant reflux episodes during one single esophageal pH monitoring study does not necessarily rule out GERD. This is especially important in patients with airway symptoms related to GERD. Tracheal irritation and respiratory symptoms may persist for weeks after a significant aspiration episode. It is possible that intermittent episodes of aspiration too infrequent to document in 1 day of 24-hour pH monitoring may produce chronic respiratory symptoms. Day-to-day variation in acid reflux is wide enough to justify scepticism when negative pH studies contradict a typical history of GERD-related symptoms.

Esophageal instillation of acid alternating with normal saline (Bernstein test) is often added to esophageal pH monitoring studies. This test is useful in evaluating the quality and severity of GERD symptoms and their temporal association with esophageal mucosal exposure to acid.

Endoscopy and Barium Swallow Studies

An inherent shortcoming of esophageal pH studies is that they only record acid exposure, which cannot be equated with mucosal damage. Esophageal pH monitoring does not take into account the resistance of the individual patient's mucosa to acid-induced injury. Mucosal integrity is assessed by endoscopy. Endoscopy is used to diagnose Barrett's esophagus and erosive esophagitis (esophageal metaplasia) because symptoms in these conditions correlate poorly with severity of esophageal injury. Endoscopy and/or barium swallow studies are also indicated to rule out structural abnormalities such as achalasia, strictures, tumors, and Zenker's diverticulum. Endoscopy is also useful in the diagnosis of duodeno-gastroesophageal reflux, which can mimic the symptoms of and often coexists with GERD.

Barium studies are used to assess the adequacy of anti-reflux mechanisms. Observing reflux of barium during fluoroscopic evaluation without the use of provoking maneuvers is of limited value because its sensitivity is estimated at 26%. The sensitivity of barium studies can be increased to 44% with the addition of reflux-eliciting maneuvers such as Valsalva, coughing, or rolling to the right. Rolling to the right while simultaneously drinking water (water-siphon test) may further increase the sensitivity of barium studies. Barium studies with associated maneuvers are less sensitive than 24-hour ambulatory esophageal pH monitoring and require a high degree of attention to technical details. The main advantages of barium studies with associated maneuvers are low cost, short examination time, and high positive predictive value (80%) (8).

Esophageal Manometry

Esophageal manometry is used to assess LES pressure and esophageal motility. A single measurement of LES pressure is abnormally low in only 4% of patients with GERD. Ineffective esophageal motility is found in 35% of patients with GERD. Other than its diagnostic value, esophageal manometry is used in selecting candidates for surgery. Patients with asthma and GERD who have normal motility, as determined by amplitude of contractions in the distal esophagus, respond better to anti-reflux surgery than do those with abnormal motility. Some surgeons also base their choice of anti-reflux surgery on esophageal manometry. Nissen fundoplication (360-deg wrap) is chosen for patients with normal peristalsis, whereas patients with peristaltic abnormalities may benefit more from a Toupet procedure (270-deg wrap).

The adoption of the therapeutic trial for the diagnosis of GERD, with gastroenterology evaluation reserved for patients who fail to respond or experience relapse of symptoms, is an accepted practice but does present certain risks. Metaplasia with columnar-lined esophagus (Barrett's esophagus) may be overlooked while GERD symptoms are being suppressed empirically. Barrett's esophagus is present in at least 10% of patients who undergo endoscopy for GERD and is diagnosed in as many as 30% of patients with erosive esophagitis. Barrett's esophagus is a serious risk factor for esophageal cancer and requires regular endoscopic evaluation. Duodeno-gastro-esophageal reflux is an additional risk factor because bile acids aggravate mucosal injury. Patients with Barrett's esophagus cannot be identified solely by their symptoms. Therefore screening endoscopy is indicated for patients with persistent symptomatic GERD (7).

Diagnosis of Other Conditions Associated with GERD and Asthma

The relationship of GERD with asthma can be compounded by other conditions that are commonly associated with either of the two diseases. These include obstructive sleep apnea, laryngospasm, and vocal cord dysfunction. Failure to recognize and treat these conditions may be a reason for poor respiratory symptom response to GERD treatment. Diagnosis of these conditions is based on sonogram, flow-volume studies, laryngoscopy, and so on.

Management of Gastroesophageal Reflux Disease

Lifestyle Changes

A stepwise approach is used for the maintenance treatment of GERD (Fig. 14-2). The goals of treatment are relief of symptoms and healing of esophagitis. Dietary and lifestyle measures are indispensable components of GERD management. Lifestyle changes include avoidance of large meals, maintaining an ideal weight, wearing loose clothing, eating the evening meal at least 3 hr before retiring, avoiding recumbency for 2 hr after a meal, and elevating the head of the bed with 6-inch blocks. The use of a foam wedge to elevate both the trunk and head is an alternative to elevation of the bed. Cessation of smoking is recommended. Carbonated drinks, alcohol, peppermint, coffee (caffeinated and decaffeinated), chocolate, and fatty acids should be avoided because they lower the LES pressure. Citrus juices, alcohol, and tomato-based products are direct esophageal irritants. Drugs lowering the LES pressure include calcium channel blockers,

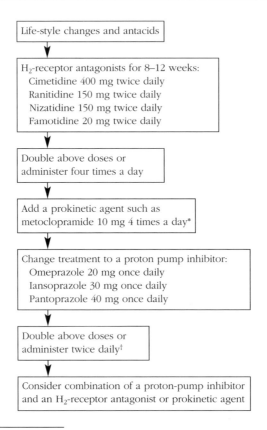

* Domperidone is used as an investigational drug, 10 mg, 15–30 minutes before meals and at bedtime.

Figure 14-2   Staging of maintenance treatment of GERD.

benzodiazepines, narcotics, nicotine, estrogen, and progesterone. Twenty percent of patients with GERD may respond to a combination of antacids and lifestyle changes, but patients with asthma are less likely to respond to lifestyle changes alone.

Pharmacotherapy

H_2-receptor antagonists may be used to control GERD. The usual initial doses are: cimetidine 800 mg twice a day, ranitidine 150 mg twice a day, nizatidine 150 mg twice a day, and famotidine 20 mg twice a day. Administration of H_2-receptor antagonists once a day or on alternate days, a practice used with success in the treatment of peptic ulcer disease, is not effective in GERD. Healing rates for erosive esophagitis approximate 50% with H_2-receptor antagonists alone. Complete esophageal healing is a prerequisite for the normalization of esophageal motility and effective acid clearance. Esophageal healing, however, may not be possible for all patients without previous restoration of normal acid clearance. Thus treatment of severe cases with H_2-receptor antagonists alone is often inadequate. Doubling the aforementioned doses or administering treatment four times a day is an option in refractory cases.

Proton-pump inhibitors have a greater antisecretory effect and esophageal healing rate than H_2-receptor antagonists. Proton-pump inhibitor therapy is indicated for patients not responding to H_2-receptor antagonists and/or prokinetic agents. Omeprazole 20 mg once a day, lansoprazole 30 mg once a day, or pantoprazole 40 mg once a day is indicated for these cases. These doses are ineffective in approximately 27% of patients who will, however, respond to doubling of the dose. Experience with pantoprazole is limited. Omeprazole doses of 80 mg/day and lansoprazole 120 mg/day have been used to control GERD with erosive esophagitis. Once treatment of erosive esophagitis has been completed, maintenance with H_2-receptor antagonists along with lifestyle changes and possibly antacids may be adequate (Case 14-3).

Prokinetic agents effective in GERD include metoclopramide and domperidone. Cisapride, a prokinetic agent now withdrawn from the US market because of its association with arrhythmias, heals esophagitis in 50% of patients. This rate is similar to the less expensive cimetidine. Domperidone has also been reported to cause QT prolongation and ventricular tachyarrhythmias. Prokinetic agents are sometimes used as an adjunct to therapy with an H_2-receptor antagonist because H_2-receptor antagonists have no effect on gastric emptying. Such combinations are often successful because they address two separate but interdependent components of GERD: acid exposure (H_2-receptor antagonist) and gastric emptying (prokinetic agent). The cost of long-term therapy can be a limiting factor.

Adverse Treatment Events and Drug Interactions

Theophylline, beta-agonists, and oral steroids decrease the LES pressure in normal subjects. In addition, theophylline increases gastric acid production, and systemic steroids delay esophageal mucosal healing. However, discontinuation of any of these agents does not result in significant improvement of reflux as documented by pH probe studies in asthmatics (2). Improvement of GERD resulting from the discontinuation of these medications is usually offset by increases in asthma symptoms that may exacerbate GERD. Inhaled corticosteroids and leukotriene inhibitors have no effect on GERD.

Prescribing GERD medication for patients with respiratory diseases requires consideration of drug interactions. The effects of cimetidine on microsomal enzyme systems result in reduction of the hepatic metabolism of theophylline. Lowering of the theophylline dose is therefore required for patients treated with cimetidine. Ranitidine variably interacts with

---

CASE 14-3   *Patient whose asthma symptoms resolve with treatment of gastroesophageal reflux disease*

An 18-year-old woman is referred for specialist evaluation for persistent nocturnal cough and dyspnea. Her cough is dry, has occurred in spells of 20 to 45 min, and has been present for 1 year at the time of her referral. The cough usually starts early in the evening but sometimes awakens her during the night. Treatment with beta-agonist inhalers has resulted in shorter and less frequent coughing/dyspnea spells but has not abolished them. Addition of an inhaled steroid has worsened her cough. There is no significant past medical history, except for acute bronchitis 1 year before presentation. She denies asthma in childhood, sinus infections, hospitalizations, and operative procedures. She is an athlete who exercises regularly and experienced no dyspnea or coughing during exercise until a year before her presentation. She denies smoking, alcohol consumption, and dietary excesses, but she admits to drinking large amounts of coffee and citrus juices. She also admits to skipping lunch often and eating large meals late at night just before going to bed in order to accommodate her busy schedule. Family history is significant for gastroesophageal reflux in her mother. Review of systems is significant for heartburn, for which she has taken H_2-receptor antagonists and antacids off and on (after the advice of her mother), but she has always discontinued them after 2 to 5 days upon relief from heartburn.

Physical examination is significant for frequent throat clearing. Upon questioning she denies having heartburn during the examination. Her peak expiratory flow rate is well above the predicted value, and pulmonary function tests are all within normal values. Rhinolaryngoscopy is normal.

Discussion

This patient was diagnosed with GERD. Beta-agonist and steroid inhalers were discontinued. She continued her H_2-receptor antagonist and was placed on a proton-pump inhibitor for 3 months. Lifestyle and dietary advice were given. Her cough/dyspnea and heartburn had resolved completely by the end of the 3-month trial. The throat clearing persisted for another 3 months. Treatment was continued with an H_2-receptor antagonist for 6 months. She did not require any asthma medication. Esophagoscopy 6 months after discontinuation of all treatment revealed satisfactory healing and no evidence of metaplasia. Repeated spirometries were normal. Follow-up visits dispelled all suspicions of asthma.

---

enzymes, and its effect on theophylline metabolism is minimal. Famotidine and nizatidine do not bind the cytochrome P450 and can be administered without adjustment of theophylline dosage. Omeprazole is metabolized via the P450 system but has no interactions with theophylline. Lansoprazole increases the clearance of theophylline by 10%, but dosage adjustment is usually not required.

Cisapride, troleandomycin, and azole antifungals such as ketoconazole, itraconazole, and clotrimazole are also metabolized via the cytochrome P450 system. Increased serum levels of cisapride carry a risk for ventricular arrhythmias. Metoclopramide can trigger extrapyramidal syndromes and is contraindicated in patients taking dopamine receptor antagonists such as phenothiazines, butyrophenones, and thioxanthenes.

Surgery

The most widely accepted indication for anti-reflux surgery in the past was the failure of medical therapy. Currently, proton-pump inhibitors provide satisfactory medical management in almost all cases, and medical failure is no longer a reason for surgical referral. Symptoms persisting despite documented adequate medical therapy are likely to have causes other than GERD (see Fig. 14-1). In fact, failure of a therapeutic trial with a proton-pump inhibitor is used by many as a predictor of poor outcome of fundoplication.

The advantage of surgery over medical treatment is that fundoplication not only removes the acid insult but also prevents fluids from refluxing into the esophagus. This makes it a preferred choice in circumstances where prevention of aspiration is a priority. Early referral for surgery is indicated for infants responding poorly to medical treatment in whom aspiration and apneas/bradycardias represent life threats. Surgery is also indicated for patients with severe GERD complications caused by aspiration (e.g., bronchiectasis, lung abscess, vocal cord ulceration). Early consideration of surgery should be given for cases where immediate prevention of aspiration is desired because of underlying conditions that place an additional burden on the integrity of the respiratory tract. Such conditions include bronchiectasis or chronic sinusitis in patients with GERD and compromised immune system, cystic fibrosis, or alpha-1 antitrypsin deficiency.

Surgery may also be indicated for financial reasons as a cost-effective alternative to medical maintenance therapy. This consideration is based on the prerequisite that surgery will provide a permanent cure. Although short-term results of open fundoplication show a success rate of 90%, long-term follow-up studies of longer than 20 years indicate that an increasing percentage of the operations do not provide permanent relief.

Many practitioners feel that in the patient with asthma, surgery should not be postponed until medical options are exhausted, and they advocate early referral for surgical treatment. In addition to the financial aspects of long-term medical management, Nissen fundoplication is more effective than ranitidine (150 mg three times a day) in improving pulmonary function in patients with asthma and GERD. Others find that omeprazole is at least as effective as fundoplication in controlling GERD and GERD-related pulmonary symptoms. Controlled studies comparing the use of proton-pump inhibitors and fundoplication are not available.

Subjects with extrinsic/allergic asthma with primarily exercise-induced asthma or asthma preceding the onset of GERD symptoms by several years are less likely to have respiratory benefits from surgery. Some surgeons use the positive response of GERD symptoms to the therapeutic trial with proton-pump inhibitors as a predictor of surgery outcome. They find this approach useful in identifying patients likely to benefit from surgery. This practice may also have a place in the evaluation of the asthmatic with GERD with respect to respiratory pathology. Therapeutic trials with proton-pump inhibitors may fail to improve asthma and may even fail to alleviate GERD symptoms. It is likely that in such patients asthma symptoms are not triggered by GERD and therefore the outcome of fundoplication may be poor for both GERD and asthma.

Laparoscopic Nissen fundoplication is being used increasingly in the management of GERD. This procedure is less invasive and is associated with lower morbidity rates than the "open" approach, which requires thoracotomy/laparotomy. Failure rates depend on the operative experience of the surgeon and may be as low as 3.5% compared with 9% to 30% for the "open" method. Failure is usually caused by slipped/misplaced, disrupted, herniated, or too tight/too long fundoplication. Improving operative techniques and increasing experience with laparoscopic revision after failure make laparoscopic fundoplication an attractive option and add to the advantages of surgical management of GERD.

Summary

Asthma and GERD contribute significantly to the pathology of each other: the physiologic changes of asthma exacerbation aggravate GERD, and GERD precipitates asthma symptoms. GERD with atypical presentation and asymptomatic GERD may account for failure of asthma treatment or unexplained deterioration of asthma control. GERD is also associated with a variety of upper airway conditions, such as sinusitis, pharyngitis, and vocal cord dysfunction, that affect respiratory function.

Because of the high prevalence of GERD among patients with asthma, detailed questioning of patients with asthma for GERD-related symptoms often leads to early diagnosis, prevents significant complications, and may limit exacerbations of asthma. Asthmatics with symptomatic GERD can be identified with a fair degree of certainty in the office setting. A therapeutic trial of acid inhibition with proton-pump inhibitors is a useful modality that allows identification of patients whose asthma may respond to treatment of GERD.

Medical treatment of GERD is effective. Asthmatics are likely to benefit from treatment with H_2-receptor antagonists, proton-pump inhibitors, prokinetic agents, antacids, or a combination of these. Staging of management and appropriate adjustments with regard to drug interactions, side effects, and cost are needed in long-term maintenance treatment. Patients whose pathology is dominated by aspiration may benefit from early referral for surgery.

■   ■   ■

Key Points

- GERD is commonly associated with asthma, occurring in 45% to 89% of patients with chronic asthma.

- Asthma precipitates acid reflux by decreasing intrathoracic pressure, and GERD in turn contributes to asthma through aspiration and neurogenic inflammation.

- Improvement in asthma symptoms follows GERD treatment in as many as 69% of patients.

- GERD may be diagnosed by resolution of symptoms with a trial of pharmacologic treatment. Other tests (e.g., endoscopy, 24-hour pH monitoring, esophageal manometry) are used for the evaluation of specific aspects of GERD pathophysiology.

- The goals of GERD treatment are relief of symptoms and healing of esophagitis. Complete esophageal healing is necessary for normalization of esophageal motility and effective acid clearance.

- Although agents used for the treatment of asthma (e.g., theophylline, beta-agonists) predispose to GERD, discontinuation of these agents does not improve reflux symptoms.

■   ■   ■

REFERENCES

1. **Theodoropoulos DS, Lockey RF, Boyce HW, Jr, Bukantz SC.** Gastroesophageal reflux in asthma: a review of pathogenesis, diagnosis and therapy. Allergy. 1999;54:651–61.

2. **Sontag SJ, O'Connell S, Khandelwal S, et al.** Most asthmatics have gastroesophageal reflux with or without bronchodilator therapy. Gastroenterology. 1990; 99:613–20.

3. **Field SK, Sutherland LR.** Does medical antireflux therapy improve asthma in asthmatics with gastroesophageal reflux? Chest. 1998;114;275–83.

4. **Herve P, Denjean A, Jian R, et al.** Intraesophageal perfusion of acid increases the bronchomotor response to methacholine and to isocapnic hyperventilation in asthmatic subjects. Am Rev Respir Dis. 1986;134:986–9.

5. **Field SK.** A critical review of the studies of the effects of simulated or real gastroesophageal reflux on pulmonary function in asthmatic adults. Chest. 1999;115:848–56.

6. **Jamieson JR, Stein HJ, DeMeester TR, et al.** Ambulatory 24-hr esophageal pH monitoring: normal values, optimal thresholds, specificity, sensitivity and reproducibility. Am J Gastroenerol. 1992;87:1102–11.

7. **Ghillebert G, Demeyere AM, Janssens J, Vantrappen G.** How well can quantitative 24-hour intraesophageal pH monitoring distinguish various degrees of reflux disease? Dig Dis Sci. 1995;40:1317–24.

8. **Thompson JK, Koehler RE, Richter JE.** Detection of gastroesophageal reflux: value of barium studies compared with 24-hr pH monitoring. Am J Roentgenol. 1994;162:621–6.

SUGGESTED READING

Beedassy A, Katz PO, Gruber A, et al. Prior sensitization of esophageal mucosa by acid reflux predisposes to reflux-induced chest pain. J Clin Gastroenterol. 2000;31:121–4.

DeVault KR, Castell DO. Guidelines for the diagnosis and treatment of gastroesophageal reflux disease: practice parameters committee of the American College of Gastroenterology. Arch Intern Med. 1995;155:2165–73.

James DE, Nijkamp FP. Neuro-immune interactions in the lung. Clin Exper Allergy. 1999;29:1309–19.

Morales TG, Sampliner RE. Barrett's esophagus: update on screening, surveillance and treatment. Arch Intern Med. 1999;159:1411–6.

Stein MR, ed. Gastroesophageal Reflux Disease and Airway Disease. New York: Marcel Dekker; 1999.

Index

Index